Comments on *Basic Skills in Statistics: A ...* *Professionals* from read...

'This publication is a fantastic resource for any h... interest in research and goes a long way to demystifying the world of statistics. It attempts to explain complex statistical concepts by applying these to practice. Packed full of useful key messages and an excellent glossary of terms, this should be an essential reference book for any budding researchers and anyone wishing to have a greater understanding of research papers.'

Monica Fletcher,
Chief Executive, National Respiratory Training Centre

'This easy to use book will open up a new world for those who have a blind spot for statistics. Using everyday examples, the authors bring to life statistical principles in a way that is relevant to clinicians and researchers alike. I will certainly be recommending it to my students, trainees and consultant colleagues.'

Professor Abdul Rashid Gatrad, OBE,
Consultant Paediatrician, Manor Hospital, Walsall

'This excellent book is based on a series of articles published in the Primary Care Respiratory Journal (www.thepcrj.org) . Not many scientific authors are capable of expressing themselves in plain English – the authors of this book have certainly achieved this. They have managed to convey the principles and to share with the reader, their very practical approach to the use of statistics in design, understanding and application in research. A book for anyone wishing to improve their understanding of evidence based medicine and those involved in research.'

Mark Levy,
Editor, Primary Care Respiratory Journal

'I found this a most enjoyable read – quite a shock for a statistics book! This is because it is much more – it explains how studies in health should be designed and interpreted as well as the statistics that should be used. It really does take the mystery away. This will help those involved in all extremes of health care research from the reader of their favourite journal, the guideline evidence reviewer right through to those designing studies. I shall be making it obligatory reading for everyone in my research team and recommending it to anyone who seriously wants to understand the papers they are reading.'

David Price,
GPIAG Professor of Primary Care Respiratory Medicine,
University of Aberdeen

Basic Skills in Statistics

A Guide for Healthcare Professionals

Adrian Cook BSc, MSc
Senior Statistician
Commission for Health Improvement

Gopalakrishnan Netuveli BSc, BDS, MDS, PhD
Post Doctoral Research Fellow
Department of Primary Health Care and General Practice
Imperial College London

Aziz Sheikh BSc, MSc, MBBS, MD, MRCP, MRCGP, DCH, DRCOG, DFFP
Professor of Primary Care Research and Development
Division of Community Health Sciences:
GP Section, University of Edinburgh;
Editorial Advisor, British Medical Journal;
Chairman, Research & Documentation Committee,
Muslim Council of Britain

CLASS HEALTH • LONDON

Printing history
First published 2004

The authors and publishers welcome feedback from the users of this book.
Please contact the publishers:
Class Publishing, Barb House, Barb Mews, London, W6 7PA, UK
Telephone: 020 7371 2119 [International +4420]
Fax: 020 7371 2878
Email: post@class.co.uk
Visit our website – www.class.co.uk

A CIP catalogue record for this book is available from the British Library

ISBN 1 85959 101 9

Edited by Carrie Walker

Designed and typeset by Martin Bristow

Illustrations by David Woodroffe

Indexed by Kathleen Lyle

Printed and bound in Great Britain
by Creative Print and Design (Wales) Ebbw Vale, Gwent

Contents

Foreword

In many medical schools, the teaching of statistics remains woefully inadequate, the same problem existing in many undergraduate courses for other healthcare professionals. Yet, more than ever, all healthcare professionals need a firm understanding of key principles of statistics. Practitioners of evidence-based care need to be able to appraise scientific papers to see whether they answer the clinical problem in question, and to assess the robustness of results presented. Clinicians wishing to audit their practice need to be able accurately to summarise and interpret their findings in order to learn whether they are providing appropriate care. In addition, an increasing number of practitioners wish to develop and conduct their own research in order to answer important clinical questions.

Most books on statistics are written for the specialist, often being full of formulae and jargon. This is unfortunate because computer programs for performing statistical tests are readily available, removing the need to perform long, complicated calculations. The users of these programs still, however, need to know the principles behind them so that they can chose correctly between the wide variety of tests and techniques available. It is refreshing, therefore, to come across a book that introduces key statistical issues in clear, uncomplicated language.

I first read the articles upon which *Basic Skills in Statistics* is based when they appeared in the *Primary Care Respiratory Journal*. The authors' clarity of thought and writing immediately impressed me. Concepts that often perplex non-researchers were presented in a plain, straightforward way. The articles rapidly became resource material for a short course that I was running on how to use data for clinical decisions. I feel sure the book will soon be found on the reading lists of other courses as well as the bookshelves of many libraries, practices and practitioners' offices. The authors are to be congratulated for providing non-experts with such a clear introduction to statistics.

Philip Hannaford,
Grampian Health Board Professor of Primary Care,
University of Aberdeen

Acknowledgements

We would like to take this opportunity to express our gratitude to Dr Mark Levy, Editor of the General Practitioner in Airways Group's *Primary Care Respiratory Journal* for permission to republish, in adapted and expanded form, our Statistical Notes series. It was the *Journal*'s editorial board who had the foresight to commission the original series of articles; we are pleased that this series proved popular with readers, many of whom might previously have had an aversion to statistics, and it is the strength and volume of the feedback that has provided the impetus for this book.

Our thanks go also to all those who commented and to our many colleagues at the General Practitioner in Airways Group and in our host institutions who so constructively commented on earlier drafts and, in so doing, have undoubtedly enhanced the quality of our work. Finally, and most importantly, we take pleasure in recording our immense debt to our wives and families, who so patiently facilitated our efforts.

Introduction

The aim of this book is to introduce healthcare professionals to basic statistical concepts. We do not claim to provide a comprehensive summary of statistics but rather hope to develop a sufficient understanding and vocabulary to enable clinicians to appraise and interpret the statistics most commonly used in research papers and, for those wishing to pursue their own research, to facilitate the discussion of their ideas with a statistician.

Although clinicians often perceive this to be an obscure and threatening discipline, the basics of statistics are really quite straightforward. At its simplest level, statistics is about summarising and presenting data in ways that accurately reflect and convey their meaning. The next main level is hypothesis-testing – the process of systematically answering a research question of importance. Typical examples of issues important to healthcare professionals include trying to ascertain whether a newly launched treatment is better than an existing drug or whether a possible risk factor, for example low birth weight, is associated with a particular outcome, such as the likelihood of developing asthma. The essence of this is to begin by assuming that the treatment or risk factor has no effect; this is sometimes referred to as the null hypothesis. The likelihood that any difference between groups has arisen by chance is then calculated. If, in a well-designed study, it is unlikely that the study groups are similar, the researcher has 'got a result' (although a 'negative' result can be just as important!). This illustrates an aspect of statistics that is often forgotten – its contribution to study design. Closely related to hypothesis-testing is estimation, whereby the researcher goes on to investigate just how different the groups under study actually are.

Through the seven chapters that follow, we will introduce issues related to data presentation (Chapters 1 and 2), the principles of hypothesis-testing (Chapter 3) and estimation (Chapter 4). Chapter 5 focuses on epidemiological and intervention study designs, and includes a discussion on the principles of undertaking sample size calculations. In Chapter 6, the penultimate chapter, we consider the role and methods of undertaking systematic reviews and meta-analyses. The final chapter touches on some of the 'nuts and bolts' of statistical issues that are important for those considering undertaking their own research projects.

Statistical jargon can sometimes be confusing so, for ease of reference, we have provided a detailed glossary of some of the most important and commonly used terms. Suggestions for further reading are also listed for those who, like us, have had their appetites whetted and wish further to pursue their interests . . .

Adrian Cook,
Gopalakrishnan Netuveli
and Aziz Sheikh

Chapter 1

Laying the foundations: measurement and probability

Key messages

- Measurement involves mapping an aspect of an object on to a scale according to specified rules.

- There are four types of measurement scale: nominal, ordinal, interval and ratio.

- Measurements generate numerical (quantitative) and categorical (qualitative) random variables.

- The insightful analysis and interpretation of statistical data are dependent on a basic appreciation of probability theory.

The building blocks of statistics

As healthcare professionals, we use both measurement and probability in our day-to-day practice. Many of the components of a routine medical examination – the taking of a patient's temperature, pulse and blood pressure, for example – are measurements. Noting features such as the presence of cyanosis and the absence of jaundice are further example of measurement, these examples underscoring the point that measurement is not confined solely to the recording of numerical data. An observation such as 'patients on oral cortico-steroids tend to put on weight' is an example of a probability statement. Descriptions of a symptom complex as 'common' or a disease as 'rare' are further examples of probability statements made in everyday practice. We will sometimes even make complex probability pronouncements, such as when we conclude that 'a

diagnosis of gallstones is likely in a fat, fair, fertile, female of forty'
with intermittent right upper quadrant abdominal pain. This last
statement is in actual fact a very succinct translation of a multiple
regression equation relating weight, skin colour, parity, age and sex
with the risk of developing cholelithiasis. These risk factors are
measured using different kinds of measurement scale, this example
thereby capturing and exemplifying the complex interrelationships
between measurement, probability and medicine.

Measurement

What does measuring entail?

Whether recording temperature or noting the presence of cyanosis,
measurement involves mapping some aspect of the object of interest
on to a scale. This operation of mapping (e.g. measuring the height of
a child) should follow some specified rules. The three most important
rules of measurement are that the:

- Scale should be unique, i.e. allow one-to-one mapping
- Measure should be meaningful
- Measure should be representative.

A practice-based example should help to illustrate the application
of these rules. Consider a primary care team wishing to study ethnic
variations in healthcare utilisation. Wishing to keep things simple for
the reception staff who will be collecting the data, they develop a
3-item scale measuring ethnicity: 1=British, 2=Asian and 3=Afro-
Caribbean. Although apparently straightforward, this is in fact a poor
measure since it fails all three of our criteria. A British-born person of
Asian descent can, for example, be classified as being both British and
Asian, so mapping is not unique. Second, defining ethnic categories
on the basis of either place of birth or the nationality the person currently holds is unlikely to be meaningful to the study of ethnicity.
Finally, such a simple scale is unlikely to represent the complex social
dynamics inherent within notions of ethnicity.

Uses of measures

There are four common uses of variables that have been measured. These are to:

- Classify objects (a child, for example, being classified as tall or short)
- Rank an object in relation to other objects
- Determine the extent of differences in attribute between two or more objects
- Find the ratio of an attribute between two or more objects.

Although measurement scales typically consist of numerical values, this need not necessarily be the case. Numerical scales do, however, have the advantage of possessing properties that allow for each of the four operations described above to be easily undertaken.

Types of measurement scale

Measurement scales can be classified according to the types of operation they allow to be undertaken. There are four types of measurement scale: nominal, ordinal, interval and ratio. These scales are mentioned in a particular order, such that each scale type includes all the properties and characteristics of the preceding ones. Nominal scales are thus the least versatile of the four, whereas ratio scales are, in contrast, extremely versatile.

Nominal scales

Nominal scales comprise labels or names that identify persons or objects according to some characteristic. To be considered as a measurement scale, labelling should follow the rule that the same label is not given to different persons/objects or that different labels should not be given to the same person/object. Two types of nominal scale can occur.

Type A: The assignment of labels to identify individuals. National

Insurance number is an example of a scale in which each individual is ascribed a unique identifier. With such a scale, the only statistic we can derive is the number of cases, i.e. the number of people with a National Insurance number.

Type B: The assignment of labels to groups of people or objects. Members of the same group will be assigned the same label. This process of assignment is usually called classification or categorisation and is based on establishing the equality of an uncategorised person or object with members of a category. It is very important to specify how this equality is established, something that is often overlooked. For example, individuals are commonly categorised as either male or female, a task that most of us believe we can perform without too much difficulty. But as studies in medical sociology have shown, these categories can have different meanings depending on whether we are interested in sex or gender. Even more confusingly, a particular individual may be assigned to a different category depending on whether we are referring to sex or gender. This example emphasises the importance of having explicit categorisation criteria and the need for consistency when categorising. Blood grouping is an example of a nominal scale with less-ambiguous categories.

Type B nominal scales have the advantage of yielding more detailed information than a simple count of the number of members in each of the categories. We can, for example, determine which of a number of categories are most commonly used for classification (i.e. the mode), or we may test the hypothesis that members of a group are unequally distributed between different categories (see Chapter 4).

These two types of nominal scale (A and B) can be considered as one and the same if we think of the type A scale as being a special case of the type B scale with a single unit in each category.

Ordinal scales

When categories in a nominal scale can be ranked and ordered, the measurement scale is described as ordinal. The Registrar General's social class grading is an example of an ordinal scale.

Ordinal scales are restricted to the use of the equality and inequality operators. That is to say that although we can use them to classify and, if necessary, arrange persons or objects according to the characteristic being studied, it is not possible to apply any arithmetical operations to them. This limitation is due to the fact that differences between adjacent ordinal measures are not necessarily the same. For example, the difference between being in social class I and social class II may not be identical to the difference between being in social classes III and IV. The inappropriate statistical manipulation and interpretation of data generated from ordinal scales can produce a great deal of confusion because of this limitation.

Responses to questions in many tests are often scored on Likert scales, individual scores being defined as having specific meanings. For example, on a 5-point scale (1–5) scores may be defined as 1 = Strongly disagree, 2 = Disagree, 3 = Neutral, 4 = Agree, and 5 = Strongly agree. Many test instruments require such scores to be summed to produce a single index. Although illegal in the mathematical sense, such transformations can nonetheless often yield useful results. The reasonable thing to do is to be cautious in interpreting the results thus derived. We would, for example, not dream about deriving 4.4 as the average social class for a group, but it might be reasonable, in certain circumstances, to have 4.4 as the mean level of agreement between 10 GPs evaluating the contents of a postgraduate lecture they had just attended.

Pursuing the example of GPs scoring of a postgraduate lecture, we can see another way in which the interpretation of summary values may not always be straightforward or indeed appropriate. Describing a mean score suggests that there is a degree of agreement between the group of GPs, but this result could conceivably have been obtained by only a few GPs strongly agreeing whereas the majority remained neutral. In such a scenario, can the mean score still be seen as an accurate reflection of GPs' views on the lecture they have just attended? More valid statistics for ordinal scales are the median and percentiles (see Chapter 2). Any method of transformation that maintains the order of the scale can be applied to ordinal scales.

Interval scales

In addition to classifying and ordering, interval scales allow us to make inferences about the differences between categories. In interval scales, numbers 1 and 3 are as equally distant as numbers 3 and 5. Adding a constant to the interval scale does not change it, and it is this property – i.e. not having an absolute zero – that is the most important limitation of this scale. The point in a measurement scale at which the characteristic of interest is absent can be considered as the 'absolute' or 'true' zero. In the interval scale, '0' need not refer to that point. By adding (or subtracting) a constant, one can change the zero point. Familiar examples of interval scales are the Fahrenheit and Celsius scales for temperature. Using either scale, we can test whether temperature differences between objects are equal, and we can transform results from one scale to another. However, '0' on the Celsius scale is not equal to '0' in Fahrenheit, both being arbitrarily set. With no anchoring point such as absolute zero, we cannot make assumptions about ratios and proportions. For example, 100°C is double 50°C on the Celsius scale, but this does not equate to a doubling on the Fahrenheit scale, on which the equivalent temperatures are 212 and 122. Most of the statistics described in this book can be used with interval scales.

Ratio scales

Most of the physical measurements we encounter are in ratio scales. Ratio scales have an absolute zero, and we are therefore able to test the equality of proportions and ratios. We would, for example, be correct to note that a son's height is half that of his father as this relationship will be retained irrespective of whether the height is measured in centimetres or inches. Such transformations between two ratio scales measuring the same attribute are achieved by multiplication by a constant. Among the commonly used measurements in medical practice, blood pressure, weight and pulse are further examples of measurements made using ratio scales. Ratio scales allow the full range of statistics that can be applied to interval scales but in addition allow more complex statistics, such as the coefficient of variation, to be derived.

Types of data

Categorical and numerical data

Measurements generate data of different types. In the four types of measurement scale described above, the nominal and ordinal scales do not necessarily require numerical representation, whereas the interval and ratio scales always need numerical labels. This fundamental distinction allows data produced from interval and ratio scales to be described as numerical or quantitative, in contrast to the categorical or qualitative data produced with nominal and ordinal scales.

Categorical data have two or more categories into one of which it is possible to place each study participant. The classification of asthma status (asthmatic or non-asthmatic) and sex (male or female) provides examples of categorical data. Ordinal variables are a subset of categorical variables in which the categories possess a clear natural ordering. The categorisation of smoking status as non-smoker, light smoker or heavy smoker is an example of ordinal categorical data.

Numerical data are either continuous or discrete. Continuous data take values anywhere on a scale; the measurement of peak expiratory flow, temperature, height and weight are common examples. Discrete data are, in contrast, limited to positive integers; the number of asthma exacerbations experienced by an individual in a year is an example of discrete information as this must always be a whole number. Both interval and ratio scales can produce continuous or discrete data.

The distinction between data types is, however, not always clear cut since numerical data may sometimes (usefully) be transformed into categorical data. For example, data on the number of cigarettes smoked per day can be treated as numerical, with typical values of between 0 and 100. Alternatively, categories of light and heavy smoking can be defined and each individual then classified as being either a non-smoker, light smoker or heavy smoker.

Variables

In research, measuring some characteristic of an object or a person produces data. Since the value of that measure varies from individual

Table 1.1 Types of random variable

Numerical	Continuous	Observations may take any value
		Usually generated from measurements
	Discrete	Observations limited to certain values
		Usually counts of an event occurring
Categorical	Nominal	Each subject placed into one of the categories
		Usually characteristic attributes of the study subjects
	Ordinal	Categories possess a clear natural ordering

to individual, the symbolic representation of those data is referred to as a variable. Measurement is always accompanied by a degree of error, which, in the absence of any other influences, is random. Variables are therefore often referred to as 'random variables'. Table 1.1 details the different types of random variables.

A dichotomous categorical variable that takes the value 1 to indicate the presence of some attribute and 0 its absence is a particularly useful type of random variable. As this scale has only two values (0 and 1), and their difference is constant, it may be considered as an interval scale. Owing to the attractive properties of this 0/1 dichotomous variable, researchers often transform more complex multiple outcome categorical variables into a series of 0/1 dichotomous variables. Such constructed dichotomous variables are called 'dummy variables'. To describe a variable with n categories, $n-1$ dummy variables are needed. The category omitted then becomes the absence of all other categories.

Random variables are subject to the laws of chance, so an understanding of statistics – the science of collecting, summarising and analysing data subject to random variation – requires a basic appreciation of probability.

Probability

Probability as a frequency

Probability can perhaps be most easily understood by considering the concept of frequency. Probability refers to the determination of the frequency of an outcome in an entire population. Suppose we have a population consisting of 2000 patients registered with a GP, 1100 of whom are male; the chance, or probability, of a patient on that GP list being male is 1100/2000=0.55. In this example, we are in the fortunate position of knowing the whole population frequency. Such detailed information is, however, often not available, in which case we are forced to resort to using smaller samples. Our estimate of the frequency of a particular outcome from a sample is termed the relative frequency. If all the outcomes of a measurement are equally possible, the probability of the outcome of interest can be calculated as 1/(number of outcomes). In the absence of any prior knowledge, it is reasonable to consider all outcomes as being equally possible, so we can calculate the probability of a patient being male as ½=0.5.

The experiment commonly associated with probability is tossing a coin. The outcome can be the coin landing as either a head or a tail, and both outcomes are considered equally probable. We can represent this probability for heads as ½ and for tails as ½. However, imperfections in the coin and differences in the way it is tossed from one time to another makes this exact probability theoretical. If we toss the coin only a small number of times, heads and tails need not come up equally. As the number of tosses increases, however, the frequency of heads and tails approaches 50% each. Table 1.2 demonstrates this point, detailing the results obtained when tossing a coin was simulated using a computer program.

Table 1.2 Frequency of 'heads' at different number of throws of coin

Number of throws	100	1 000	10 000	100 000	1 000 000
Frequency	0.49	0.522	0.4948	0.499 36	0.499 567

The whole table represent 1 111 100 throws, and the frequency of heads in this sample was 0.499 525, with an error of only − 0.000 475 from the expected frequency (0.5).

Properties of probability

Probability has three key properties:

- It is bound within the interval between 0 and 1
- Outcomes should be mutually exclusive
- Events should be independent.

In a trial of 100 throws, if there were no heads, the probability would be 0/100=0, and if all the throws turned up as heads, the probability would be be 100/100=1. Probability is therefore bound within these limits.

If the outcomes are not mutually exclusive, 0 and 1 will not bind the probability. Consider what happens if the coin landing on its edge is categorised as both head and tail. In a trial of 100 throws, heads alone, tails alone and both heads and tails occur 40, 40 and 20 times respectively. Now heads has occurred a total of 60 times, so the probability of heads is 0.6. Similarly, the probability for tails is also 0.6. From this, it seems that in this trial of 100 throws, we can get a head or a tail 120 times, i.e. a probability of 1.2!

Frequency cannot be used to define probability in the absence of the third property, i.e. independence. Suppose heads and tails always alternate. In this case, after a trial of 100 tosses, the frequency of heads is 50 and that of tails also 50. The probability of heads or tails is not, however, 0.5 each because, after the first toss, we know the outcomes of all subsequent throws. In this case, the probability is not defined by the frequencies of outcome.

In the case of mutually exclusive outcomes, adding the probabilities of each outcome together gives the probability of getting one or the other outcome. When two events are independent, the probability of both occurring is the product of their individual probabilities.

Probability distribution

We can calculate the probabilities of all possible outcomes for 10 tosses of a coin, which will range from 0 heads to 10 heads. Figure 1.1 shows the distribution of these probabilities; it can be seen that 5 heads is the most likely result, whereas 0 or 10 heads is possible but extremely unlikely. As these probabilities are calculated using the binomial expansion (i.e. two mutually exclusive outcomes), this is called the binomial distribution. The binomial probability distribution describes the number of successes (the outcome of interest) in n trials, each success having a probability of P; n and P are called the parameters of the binomial distribution. In Figure 1.1, n is equal to 10 (10 tosses), and P is equal to 0.5 (the probability of a head). Using other examples with different values of n and P, the distribution will also change, generating a family of binomial distributions.

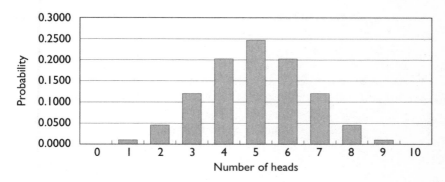

Figure 1.1 Binomial distribution with $n = 10$ and $P = 0.5$

Other distributions

There are a number of other distributions that data can follow, one of the most important of which, for categorical health-related outcomes, is the Poisson distribution. This is usually used with counts of events in a specified interval of time. The number of patients admitted per week or number of deaths per month will follow the Poisson probability distribution. The interval need not be restricted to a temporal scale. The number of accidents per kilometre of a highway will also follow the Poisson probability distribution. The Poisson distribution has only one parameter, usually represented as λ, which is equal to the average of the counts.

For continuous variables, the most common probability distribution is the normal distribution, which has been described as the most important distribution in statistics. This distribution will be discussed in more detail in the next chapter.

Summary

Knowledge of the rules and scales of measurement and an appreciation of probability theory underpin the intelligent use of statistics. Measurement requires the scale that is used to be unique, meaningful and representative. Measurements help to classify, order and compare aspects of objects. Measurement scales can be nominal, ordinal, interval or ratio scales. Because measurement is always accompanied by random errors, the symbolic representation of data produced by measurement is described as a random variable.

In this chapter, we have defined probability as a frequency that is bound by the interval 0 to 1. Other key features of probability are that outcomes are mutually exclusive and independent. The probability distribution is formed by the probabilities of all possible outcomes. Binomial, Poisson and normal are the most commonly observed probability distributions in health-orientated outcomes.

Chapter 2

Description
of a single variable

Key messages

■ Descriptive statistics allow important information about data to be conveyed in a concise manner.

■ Categorical variables can be summarised using counts and percentages.

■ Discrete numerical variables can be summarised using the mode and median as measures of location, and ranges and percentiles as measures of dispersion.

■ Normally distributed numerical variables should be summarised using the mean and standard deviation.

■ Non-normally distributed numerical variables should usually be summarised with the median and a measure of range.

Minimum information needed to describe a variable

What is the minimum information required to describe a variable such as weight? Consider the case in which the variable represents a measurement from a single individual. We will know everything about that variable if we know its value. If, however, we have weights on a group of 15 people, how do we meaningfully summarise this information? This is the realm of descriptive statistics (sometimes also referred to as summary statistics).

Descriptive statistics are widely used by researchers to summarise results in a concise yet intelligible manner. These summary statistics should provide sufficient information to allow distributions of important variables to be visualised, thereby facilitating the generation of a clear mental picture of the group being studied. Summary statistics must be selected with care, taking into consideration both the type and distribution of a variable. The different types of variables were described in Chapter 1.

Distributions of variables

Categorical variables

In the case of a nominal variable (such as blood group), the distribution of the variable is given by the frequency with which different possible values of the variable occur in the data. Figure 2.1 is a bar chart representing the distribution of participants in a blood donation campaign according to their ABO blood group. The height of the bar represents the frequency. In a bar chart, the bars should all be the same width and should not touch one another. Only one axis of the bar chart (i.e. the axis showing the frequency) has a scale; the other axis describes the categories under study.

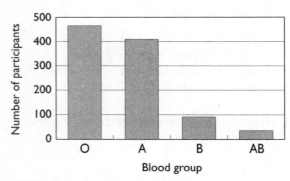

Figure 2.1 Bar chart displaying the frequency distribution of the number of participants in a blood donation drive according to their blood group ($n = 1000$)

When looking at Figure 2.1 from left to right, the frequencies appear to show a trend. It is important to remember that this has no interpretive meaning since we can, with no loss of information, shuffle the order in which categories are presented. On the other hand, Figure 2.2 displays the distribution of minor childhood accidents

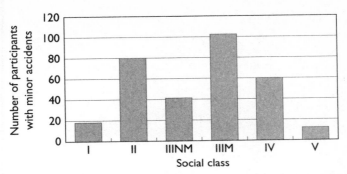

Figure 2.2 Bar chart showing the distribution of children who had a minor accident in the previous 4 weeks by social class ($n=312$)

during the previous 4 weeks by social class; in this example, there is an ordinal scale on the x-axis, and we may therefore attempt to draw conclusions regarding trends. Do you think a trend exists here?

Numerical variables

With a numerical variable, this strategy of representing distributions is not possible. The number of unique values may be so large that the frequency distribution would look like the raw data themselves. One solution is to group data into intervals on the measuring scale. Such intervals are usually referred to as 'bins' or class intervals. The bins need not be of equal size. Figure 2.3, where the intervals are equal, represents the distribution of body mass index in elderly people. This figure is called a histogram.

There are important differences between a histogram and a bar chart. In a bar chart, the height of the column represents the frequency, whereas in a histogram the frequency is represented by the area of the column. The scale on the y-axis then represents the frequency density, or frequency per unit interval. If all the intervals are the same width, the height of the histogram bars are comparable, otherwise they are not. The x-axis is a scale, so segments of equal length are equal. In a histogram, the limits of class intervals must not overlap. There are no gaps between the columns; any interval for which there are no observations will still be represented in the chart.

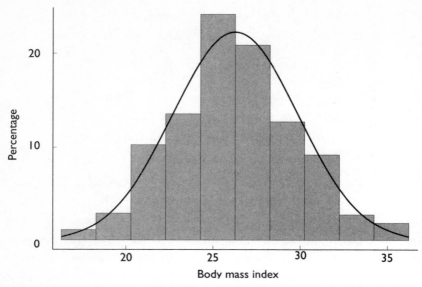

Figure 2.3 Histogram showing body mass index of British men over 65 years of age
(*n*=553)

Data			Stem and leaf	
0.3	4.9	7.9	**0**	3
1.3	4.9	8.1	**1**	34
1.4	5.5	8.4	**2**	9
2.9	5.6	8.7	**3**	02
3.0	6.1	9.9	**4**	146899
3.2	6.2		**5**	56
4.1	7.3		**6**	12
4.4	7.5		**7**	35689
4.6	7.6		**8**	147
4.8	7.8		**9**	9

Figure 2.4 Example of a stem and leaf plot displaying
25 randomly generated numbers

A further way to display data clearly is the stem and leaf plot; this is an acceptable alternative to the histogram since it allows the structure of the data to be clearly visualised. A stem and leaf plot for 25 randomly generated numbers is displayed in Figure 2.4. The first digit represents the stem, and the leaf units are 0.1. This is a true 'back of an envelope' method for visually representing data that can easily be produced by hand for small datasets.

Probability distribution function for a numerical continuous variable

Numerical variables in which the variable can take any value no matter how small the interval are known as continuous variables (see Chapter 1). There are an infinite number of possible outcomes. As a result of this, the probability of having any particular value on the continuous scale is zero. It is, however, possible to estimate the probability of a value for the particular variable falling within an interval on the scale. For example, the probability of a person chosen at random being exactly 1.735 m tall is extremely low, but the probability of their being between 1.73 and 1.74 m tall is much greater.

Using the idea that probability is the relative frequency from a large number of trials, one may try to find the probability by carrying out a large number of observations. As the number of observations increases, the bin size on the histogram becomes narrower, and the 'steps' on the top of the columns approach a smooth curve. It was mentioned earlier that, in a histogram, the area of the column represents the frequency, and the scale on the y-axis is the frequency density. In the case of a curve, the area under the curve can be determined from the equation of the curve. Now, the probability that a random variable will fall into a certain class interval is equal to the area under the curve for that class interval. If our observations include the whole population, the relative frequency is the same as the probability, and the curve is known as the probability density function. As the total area under the probability density function represents the total probability, it is equal to 1.

It is often not possible to determine the shape of the probability distribution curve, and in such situations it is generally assumed that it follows some known mathematical distribution. Thus, in Figure 2.3

above, the body mass index is assumed to follow the theoretical curve superimposed on the histogram. This symmetrical, bell-shaped curve is the 'normal' curve and is the basis of most of the statistics used in medical sciences. The parameters of the normal curve are the mean (μ) and a measure of the dispersion of data known as the variance (σ^2). In Figure 2.3, applying the mean and variance calculated from the observed data produces the normal curve.

When $\mu = 0$ and $\sigma^2 = 1$, the normal curve is known as a standard normal curve. Any normally distributed dataset can be transformed to a standard normal distribution by taking each observation in turn, subtracting the mean and dividing by the standard deviation (square root of variance). At a danger of running beyond the scope of this book, it is interesting to note that it is the ability to perform this transformation that explains the usefulness of the normal distribution, since we need to know in detail the properties of only a single distribution. In comparison, the properties of other distributions such as the binomial and Poisson distributions change with the parameter values, so in practice they are frequently replaced with a normal approximation.

Summarising data

Categorical variables

Data are usually presented as the number of subjects, together with their percentages, in each category. If there are many categories, some containing few subjects, merging categories may simplify presentation. Consider a symptom variable with four ordered categories: none, mild, moderate or severe. It may be that most subjects fall into one of the two extreme categories. With such data, the main features are perhaps best communicated by merging the middle two groups into a new category of 'some symptoms', and presenting numbers and percentages in the three groups.

Discrete numerical variables

Discrete numerical variables can be summarised using the mode and median as measures of location, and ranges and percentiles as measures of dispersion. Although it may be valid in some cases to add and average a count, this is not always appropriate as this can lead to statistics that are difficult to interpret. For example, a statement such as 'children with an upper respiratory tract infection experience pyrexia for an average of 3.5 days' might be meaningful, whereas a similar statement, such as 'GPs see an average of 17.5 patients during morning surgery', is not. Although one can imagine fractions of a day, fractions of a person are difficult to comprehend. Even then, the first statement about the number of days of pyrexia is misleading since it suggests a precision in measurement that in reality never existed. Where count data have to be summarised into an average, enlarging the denominator can in some instances solve the problem of the inappropriate fraction. It is for this reason that vital statistics data are typically reported for a large number, such as 100 000 people. The measure of dispersion most frequently associated with the mean is the standard deviation; this may, however, not be appropriate to use with discrete variables as count data often fail to satisfy the assumptions of normality.

Continuous numerical variables

Data are summarised by an average value together with a measure of how far observations are spread out around this value. The best-known averages are the mean and the median, whereas the most widely used measures of dispersion are the standard deviation and the interquartile range. The choice of which average to use, and which measure of dispersion, depends on whether the data are normally distributed. Figure 2.3 above is an example of data that are normally distributed; the symmetrical, bell-shaped curve is characteristic.

Whether data are normally distributed can often be ascertained using histograms, as in the example in Figure 2.3. Formal tests of normality, such as that of Shapiro–Wilk, are also available with most statistical packages. Determining whether the data in a small sample are normally distributed can be difficult as the shape of the distribution may not be apparent from a histogram and the Shapiro–Wilk test may have insufficient power to detect a departure from normality. Treating data as 'not normal' is the safest approach in such situations.

For normally distributed data, the mean and standard deviation are the usual parameters since they use all the data and have other useful properties. They become misleading, however, for non-normal data, which are either skewed or contain a small number of highly unusual observations (often known as 'outliers'). For such data, the median is a more appropriate average and the interquartile range a better indicator of dispersion.

Figure 2.5 shows the distribution of daily air pollutant levels (PM_{10}) over 3 years in Santiago, Chile. The concentration of PM_{10} was between 50 and $100 \mu g/m^3$ on almost half the days, whereas the level on over 90% of the days exceeded the European target of $50 \mu g/m^3$. The distribution is positively skewed, very high concentrations being noted on occasions.

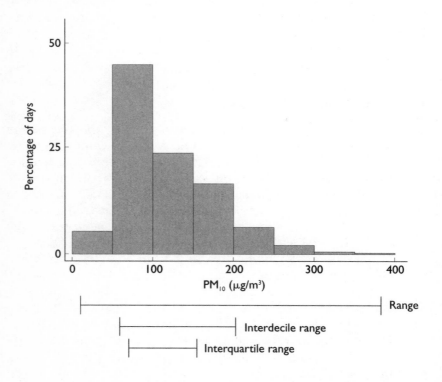

Figure 2.5 Daily particulate (PM_{10}) levels, Santiago, Chile (1992–94)

The data show why the mean is a poor indicator of location for skewed data. The mean concentration is $117\,\mu g/m^3$, whereas the median is $99.8\,\mu g/m^3 - 15\%$ lower. This difference occurs as a result of the mean being pulled upwards by the high levels in the right tail of the distribution. The magnitude of the effect depends on the degree of skewness, highly skewed data producing the greatest discrepancies. Outlying observations have a similar effect, pulling the value of the mean towards them.

When the mean is a poor indicator of location, the standard deviation should not be used since it is a measure of variation around the mean. Better indicators of dispersion are the interquartile and interdecile ranges. These give a measure of variability as well as some indication of the level of skewness. The absolute range is also suitable for skewed data but should not be used for data containing outliers. It is unusual, although on occasions informative, to present more than one range.

Returning to Figure 2.5, the data have an absolute range of $19-380\,\mu g/m^3$, an interdecile range of $59-197\,\mu g/m^3$ and an inter-quartile range of $74-152\,\mu g/m^3$. From the median and the interdecile range, it is possible to visualise the data as being skewed in their distribution, with a peak at $100\,\mu g/m^3$ and 80% of observations lying between 60 and $200\,\mu g/m^3$. The interdecile range is therefore the most informative measure of dispersion in this instance.

In Box 2.1, the various descriptive statistics for continuous variables are given.

When not to summarise

Data with more than one peak

Data cannot always be usefully summarised. For a variable with more than one peak in the distribution, both the mean and median can be very misleading. Such situations are rare but do emphasise the importance of plotting variables before summarising data.

Figure 2.6 shows the scores of subjects given a quality of life questionnaire (Euroquol). The distribution is bimodal, having two distinct peaks. The mean and median are 0.48 and 0.53 respectively.

Box 2.1 Descriptive statistics for a continuous variable

A continuous variable is described using its location, spread, and shape.

1. Measures of location:

   • **Mean** is the average value

   • **Median** is the middle point of the ordered data

   • **Mode** is the most common value observed.

2. Measures of scale or spread:

   • **Range** refers to the difference between the maximum value and the minimum value in the data

   • **Variance** is the average of the squares of the differences between the mean and each observation. For finding the average, we do not use the number of observations but the number of degrees of freedom, which is one less than the number of observations

   • **Standard deviation** is the square root of the variance.

3. Measures of shape:

   • **Skewness** refers to the degree of asymmetry of the distribution of the variable. The normal distribution has zero skewness

   • **Kurtosis** refers to the 'peakedness' of the distribution. The standard normal distribution has a kurtosis of 3.

Both values lie in the group of scores to the right, and both fail meaningfully to describe the observed data. These data can be described in detail only by showing the figure. An alternative approach, and one normally used with data from this particular questionnaire, is to categorise subjects into 'cases' and 'non-cases', 'cases' being the group to the left of the divide with the lower quality of life scores. Techniques appropriate to categorical data are then used.

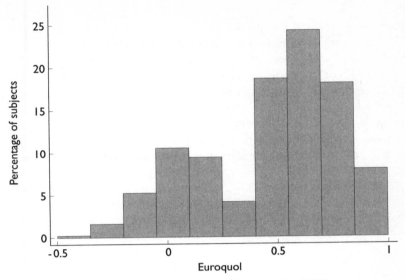

Figure 2.6 Euroquol quality of life scores ($n=1811$)

Pointers to poor summary statistics

The inappropriate use of means is a common mistake. A suspicion of skewed data should be aroused if the standard deviation is greater than the mean for a variable limited to positive values, such as age or exposure (e.g. pollen count). In such cases, the median and a measure of range would provide a more accurate summary.

It is also worrying to see a variable summarised by the mean and range. If the data are not normally distributed, the mean will usually lie some distance from the centre of the range, and the median will be more appropriate. If the mean is appropriate, the standard deviation is the best measure of dispersion, remembering that the range can still be estimated by adding and subtracting three standard deviations to the mean.

Summary

Descriptive statistics should summarise results in a concise yet intelligible manner. The type and distribution of variable affects the choice of descriptive statistics employed. Whereas categorical data can often be graphically represented by bar charts, numerical data are often visually represented using histograms and stem and leaf plots. Categorical variables are described as numbers and percentages in each category. Continuous variables can be summarised using measures of location (mean, median and mode), spread (range, variance and standard deviation) and shape (skewness and kurtosis). Summarising data is, however, not always useful and can on occasions be misleading; when reading and interpreting papers, it is therefore important to be aware of inappropriate attempts at summarising data.

Chapter 3

Linking two variables

Key messages

■ Two variables may be unrelated or related. For related
variables, the important question is whether this relationship
is a chance finding, spurious (as a result of confounding),
simply an association or a causal relationship.

■ Determining the extent of the correlation between two
continuous outcomes allows the relationship between these
variables to be assessed.

■ Contingency tables allow the strength of association between
two categorical variables to be ascertained.

■ Odds ratios and relative risks are both widely used when
summarising results. Their strength lies in the fact that they
are unaffected by changes in baseline prevalence and are
therefore 'portable'. Their major drawback, however, is that
these are relative measures and therefore difficult to interpret
in a clinical context.

■ The number-needed-to-treat and number-needed-to-harm
are derived from absolute measures of risk and are easier to
interpret clinically. These measures are now widely reported
when discussing the effectiveness and safety profile of
interventions, serving an important role in bridging the gap
between research findings and understanding their clinical
significance.

Univariate, bivariate and multivariate statistics

In the context of research, it is unusual to measure only a single aspect of an object or a person. More typically, researchers measure two or more variables in an attempt to establish whether or not a relationship exists between them. Statistical techniques dealing with a single variable are called univariate. In the previous chapter, we described univariate descriptive statistics, and the next chapter will focus on some of the inferences it is possible to make about single variables. In this chapter, we discuss bivariate statistics. Bivariate techniques such as correlation and simple regression techniques allow the identification and description of the relationships that exist between two variables. Multivariate techniques such as multiple regression use two or more variables and thus allow the analysis of more complex relationships. Although important, these techniques fall beyond the scope of this book.

Association and causation

We link two variables for the purpose of testing whether one of them influences the other. The extent of influence may vary very considerably, and we may try to show that a causal relationship exists between

---

Box 3.1 Bradford Hill's criteria for assessing causality

- **Strength** – A strong association is more likely to be causal than a weak one

- **Consistency** – A causal association should be observed in different populations at different times

- **Temporality** – The cause should precede the effect; in some cases, this may be extended such that removing a cause subsequently removes an effect

- **Gradient** – The existence of a unidirectional dose–response curve

- **Plausibility** – A hypothesis should be biologically plausible

- **Coherence** – A cause and effect relationship should not conflict with what is known to be true.

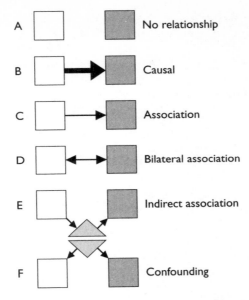

Figure 3.1 Types of relationship that can occur between two variables

the two variables. In reality, it is very unlikely that a single statistical analysis will be strong enough to satisfy the demanding criteria for determining a causal relationship that have been described by Sir Austin Bradford Hill and others (Box 3.1).

The relationship is often more accurately described simply as an association between the two variables, with no claims being made about causality. Two variables are associated if knowledge about one tells us something about the other. Figure 3.1 details the main types of relationship that can exist between two variables.

Relationship between two continuous variables

The first step in establishing a relationship between two continuous variables is to examine them together graphically. The graph used is a scatter plot in which one axis is a scale based on one variable and the other is a scale based on the other variable. Each pair of variables is represented by a dot on the graph, which is scattered (hence the name) on the plane bound by the two axes. Figure 3.2 shows three

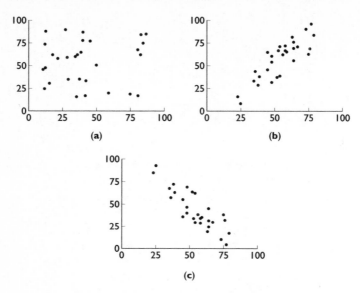

Figure 3.2 Some typical scatter plots
(a) No correlation; (b) Positive correlation; (c) Negative correlation

scatter plots: in (a), the dots are scattered without any obvious pattern; in (b), a pattern is clearly visible whereby variables on the x- and y-axes change in the same direction; and in (c), there is again a pattern, but the nature of the relationship is reversed. Expressed in a different way, we can say that there is no obvious correlation between the variables in (a) but that a correlation does appear to exist in (b) and (c), this correlation being positive in (b) and negative in (c).

Correlation coefficients

The numerical value ascribed to these relationships is the correlation coefficient, its value ranging between +1 (a perfect positive correlation) and −1 (a perfect negative correlation). Pearson's and Spearman's are the two best-known correlation coefficients. Of the two, Pearson's product–moment correlation coefficient is the most widely used, to the extent that it has now become the default. It must nevertheless be used with care as it is sensitive to deviations from normality, as might be the case if there were a number of outliers.

The Spearman correlation coefficient uses only the ranking of data, rather than their numerical values, and is therefore more suitable if only ordinal data are available. Its use might also be appropriate with continuous data that are non-normally distributed. Normality can easily be visualised using a scatter plot, in which normal data present the typical elliptical distribution seen in Figure 3.2(b) and (c).

With the correlation coefficient, the +/− sign indicates the direction of the association, a positive correlation meaning that high values of one variable are associated with high values of the other. A positive correlation exists between height and weight, for example. Conversely, when high values of one variable usually mean low values of the other (as is the case in the relationship between obesity and physical activity), the correlation will be negative.

The numerical value of the Pearson product–moment correlation coefficient (r) indicates the strength of the association, a value close to +1 or −1 indicating a strong association. In Figure 3.2(a), where there is no correlation, r is just 0.06. In Figure 3.2(b) and (c), the coefficients are respectively +0.85 and −0.85, indicating strong positive and negative correlations. When the relationship is absolutely linear, r will be +1 or −1, the sign depending on the nature of the relationship, as described above.

It is possible to calculate a valid correlation coefficient for any two variables that have a linear relationship. A significance test can then be carried out to establish how likely it is that the correlation has arisen by chance or, to express it more technically, to determine whether the correlation coefficient is significantly different from 0. To conduct a significance test, it is, however, important that another criterion is satisfied, namely that at least one of the variables should be normally distributed. Note, however, that both variables need to be normally distributed in order to calculate valid confidence intervals. Significance tests and confidence intervals are discussed in more detail in the next chapter.

Inappropriate uses of correlation coefficients

In addition to the problems related to normally distributed data, correlation coefficients can be misused in other ways. Detailed below are some of the most common ways in which such misuse tends to occur:

- When variables are repeatedly measured over a period of time, time trends can lead to spurious relationships between the variables

- Violating the assumption of random samples can lead to the calculation of invalid correlation coefficients

- Correlating the difference between two measurements to one of them leads to error. This typically occurs in the context of attempting to correlate pre-test values to the difference between pre-test and post-test scores. Since pre-test values figure in both variables, a correlation is only to be expected

- Correlation coefficients are often reported as a measure of agreement between methods of measurement whereas they are in reality only a measure of association. For example, if one variable was always approximately twice the value of the other, correlation would be high but agreement would be low.

Interpreting correlation coefficients

The clinical interpretation of the correlation coefficient is not always straightforward. However, through a relatively simple arithmetic step – calculating the square of the correlation coefficient – it is possible to obtain a clinically meaningful appreciation of the relationship that exists between two related variables. This point is perhaps best illustrated with an example.

There are many different ways of measuring lung function, peak expiratory flow (PEF) and forced expiratory volume in 1 second (FEV_1) being two of the most commonly used techniques. Whereas the former is simple, involving nothing more than a hand-held device, the latter requires more sophisticated equipment and is usually performed only under the direct supervision of a clinician. As well as the obvious practical differences in obtaining valid measures, it is important to be aware that the two approaches measure different aspects of lung function. Despite these differences, it may be interesting to see how they compare and look at the strength of the relationship (if any) that exists between the two.

Consider a study that explored this very question in a group of 61 adults and found a 'highly positive correlation of $r = 0.95$'; the authors reported that this was a statistically significant relationship with P<0.001. Precisely what constitutes a 'highly positive correlation' is, however, subjective since the correlation coefficient is a dimensionless quantity. The square of the correlation coefficient does, however, have a formal meaning, $100r^2$ being the percentage of variation in one variable 'explained' by the variation in the other. So, in this example, $(0.95)^2 = 0.90$, which indicates that 90% of the variation seen in PEF can be 'explained' by the variation in FEV_1.

Another way to interpret correlation coefficients is to compare a number of them with each another. Consider a study of 66 primary care groups in London in which the authors investigated the relationship between socio-economic factors and hospital admission rate for asthma. The analysis used socio-economic information obtained from census data and National Health Service hospital admissions data. The percentage of households without central heating was found to be more strongly associated with admission rate ($r=0.46$) than was either unemployment ($r=0.15$) or car ownership ($r=0.11$); the strongest inverse correlation was with the number of people educated to at least A level standard ($r=-0.41$).

Linear regression

In addition to being able to make a statement that two variables are correlated, it would be useful if we could predict the value of one variable from the other. The variable being predicted is by convention known as the 'dependent variable' and denoted by y, whereas the variable used for prediction is described as the 'independent variable' and is denoted by x. The relationship between the two can be summarised using the following equation for a straight line: $y = bx + a$, where b is the slope, equal to the change in y per unit change in x, and a is a constant representing the point at which the line will intercept the y-axis. Once the values for a and b have been established, it is possible to predict y from x.

When our prediction is perfect, all the data points will lie on the line. The distance of a point from the line therefore represents how much error was involved in the prediction. The problem is to find the best line, and this is done by selecting a and b in such a way that errors are minimised. We do this by the method of least squares, which refers to a process of minimising the sum of the squares of deviations from the line.

It should be noted that the values for the slope and intercept will change if x and y are swapped and we use y to predict x. The Pearson product–moment correlation coefficient is the geometrical mean of the two slopes: $r = \sqrt{b_{yx} b_{xy}}$, where b_{yx} is the slope when y is predicted from x, and b_{xy} is the slope when x is predicted from y.

This process of line-fitting is called regression, and although this has currently taken prominence over presenting simple correlation coefficients, it is important to be aware that certain assumptions need to be satisfied before attempting regression. The dependent variable should be independent, normally distributed and exhibit constant variance over the range of the independent variable (homogeneity). Furthermore, the two variables should be linearly related. On the other hand, the predictor variable need neither be normal nor from a random sample. Regression can thus be used to show the strength of the relationship in cases in which the Pearson product–moment correlation, which requires both variables to be normally distributed, cannot be used.

Relationship between two categorical variables

The first step in examining the relationship between two categorical variables is cross-tabulation, which is equivalent to the use of the scatter plot. Cross-tabulation refers to a table of frequencies, the columns being defined by categories of one variable, and the rows being defined by those of the other (Table 3.1). The intersection of a column and a row forms a cell into which is placed the count of the objects or persons who have characteristics defined by both the column and row categories. The bottom-right cell of the table will

Table 3.1 2×2 Contingency table

	Column 1	Column 2	Total
Row 1	a	b	a+b
Row 2	c	d	c+d
Total	a+c	b+d	a+b+c+d

display the total sample size. The marginal totals refer to the sum of frequencies in the columns and rows. Cross-tabulations are also sometimes known as contingency tables. The categories in the variables are independent and mutually exclusive.

Correlation between two binary variables

The correlation between two binary variables is given by the phi coefficient (ϕ). It is calculated as:

$$(\phi) = \frac{ad - bc}{\sqrt{(a+c)(b+d)(c+d)(a+b)}}$$

This will be numerically equal to Pearson product–moment correlation calculated using 0 and 1 as outcomes for both variables.

Assessing risk

A common use of a 2×2 contingency table is in assessing risk after exposure. In this case, relationships are expressed not in terms of correlations but as measures of probabilities. These are important concepts in the context of healthcare provision, and we begin this discussion by defining risk and odds, the two basic measures of disease probability. We then show how the effect of a disease risk factor, or of a treatment, can be measured using the relative risk (RR) or the odds ratio (OR). Finally, we discuss the 'number-needed-to-treat' (NNT), a measure derived from the relative risk, which has gained popularity because of its clinical usefulness.

Risk and odds

The probability of an individual becoming diseased is commonly referred to as the risk of an adverse outcome. For example, in a survey of four factories using acid anhydrides, workers were asked about respiratory problems beginning after the start of employment. Respiratory symptoms were reported by 34 of the 401 subjects, the risk therefore being 34/401=0.085, or 8.5%. In other words, among 100 factory workers exposed to acid anhydrides, 8 or 9 would be expected to develop respiratory symptoms.

The concept of odds is familiar to gamblers as the ratio between amounts at stake in a bet, an odds of 4:1 meaning that if one party stakes £4, the other stakes £1, and the winner takes the whole £5. The odds of disease refers to the ratio between the probability of disease and the probability of no disease. From surveys, the number of cases divided by the number of non-cases can estimate this. Returning to the above example, the odds of a factory worker exposed to acid anhydrides developing respiratory symptoms is $34/367 = 0.093$, slightly higher than the risk.

Rare diseases yield similar risk and odds since the number of non-cases is close to the number of subjects. For common diseases, the risk and odds can differ greatly, and it is therefore important in such situations to differentiate between the two.

Relative risk and odds ratio

The workers in the example above were employed at four different factories, the second factory being known to use large amounts of trimellitic anhydride (TMA). To investigate the relative danger of this particular chemical, the risk or odds of workers at factory 2 can be compared with that of workers at the other factories. Workers at the other factories are referred to as 'unexposed', and their risk or odds is referred to as 'baseline'. Investigations of treatment effects can be made in similar fashion by comparing disease probability in treated and untreated patients.

The relative risk compares the risk of exposed and unexposed subjects, whereas the odds ratio compares odds. A relative risk or odds ratio greater than 1 indicates an exposure to be harmful, while a beneficial exposure has a value less than 1. Thus, a relative risk of 1.2 indicates that people exposed to the risk factor of interest (TMA in this example) are 20% more likely to be diseased; similarly, a relative risk of 1.4 means that they are 40% more likely to be diseased. An odds ratio of 1.2 means that the odds of disease is 20% higher in people exposed to TMA than those not exposed to TMA.

Using the data in Table 3.2, we can calculate that the risk to workers in the factory of interest is $13/116 = 0.11$, compared with an 'unexposed' risk of $21/285 = 0.07$. The relative risk is therefore $0.11/0.07 = 1.52$; i.e. workers exposed to TMA are about 50% more

Table 3.2 Work-related respiratory symptoms, by TMA exposure

	Work-related respiratory symptoms		
	Yes	No	*Total*
Exposed	13	103	116
Not exposed	21	264	285
Total	34	367	401

likely to develop respiratory symptoms than workers exposed to other anhydrides. A similar calculation gives an odds ratio of 1.59, slightly higher than the relative risk.

Comparing relative risks and odds ratios

Relative risk is intuitively easier to understand than the odds ratio, and it is for this reason often regarded as the better of the two measures from a practitioners' viewpoint. The odds ratio can be regarded as an estimate of the relative risk when disease risk is low in both groups, say 20% or less. This approximation worsens as baseline risk or effect size increases.

Odds ratios are, however, widely used because they have mathematical advantages. They are thus commonly used in multivariate analyses, when effect estimates need to be adjusted for factors such as age, which may differ between the two groups. They are also used to analyse case-control studies, an epidemiological study design that retrospectively compares 'cases' of disease with healthy 'controls' (see Chapter 5).

The relative risk and odds ratio are both relative measures of effect and are as such unaffected by changes in baseline risk. In other words, studies carried out in different regions with different disease levels should give the same result, and it is in this 'portability' that the great strength of these relative measures lies. Their downside, however, is that they give no indication of just how many people are affected. For a given relative risk, more cases will occur if the associated disease is common than if it is rare. Understanding the implications of relative risks and odds ratios in public health terms therefore requires baseline risk to be considered.

Number-needed-to-treat

The number-needed-to-treat combines the relative risk and baseline risk into a single clinically meaningful statistic. 'Number-needed-to-treat' refers to the number of patients requiring treatment for one extra successful outcome. In terms of risk factors, it represents the number of people who must be removed from exposure to prevent one case of the disease. Problems can occur when calculating confidence intervals for the number-needed-to-treat, so to overcome this, the number-needed-to-benefit (NNTB) and the number-needed-to-harm (NNTH) have been developed.

Data from a clinical trial of smoking cessation are presented in Table 3.3. Participants received nicotine patches and either a nicotine nasal spray or a placebo spray for 1 year. Six years later, 16.1% of those given an active spray were still abstaining from smoking, compared with 8.4% of the placebo group. From the placebo group, the baseline 'risk' of stopping is 0.084. For those receiving nicotine spray, the relative risk is $0.161/0.084=1.92$; i.e. they are almost twice as likely to succeed. The number-needed-to-treat is 13, calculated from the formula given in Table 3.4; of 13 patients receiving a nicotine nasal spray in addition to a patch, one is expected to give up smoking who would not otherwise have done so.

The number-needed-to-treat is now frequently reported in trial results. When not given, it can be calculated from the relative risk and

Table 3.3 Percentages smoking at 6 year follow-up, by treatment group

	Smoking status ($n=237$)	
	No	Yes
	% (n)	% (n)
Patch and nicotine spray	16.1 (19)	83.9 (99)
Patch and placebo spray	8.4 (10)	91.6 (109)

Table 3.4 Key definitions

Measure	Definition
Risk	Number of cases / number of subjects
Odds	Number of cases / number of non-cases
Relative risk (RR)	Risk in exposed / risk in unexposed
Odds ratio (OR)	Odds in exposed / odds in unexposed
Number-needed-to-treat (NNT)	1 / (Risk in unexposed − risk in unexposed)

baseline risk. The odds ratio may be used in place of the relative risk when the risk in both groups is low.

Summary

Two variables may be related causally or, more commonly, non-causally. Stringent criteria need to be applied before accepting causation. Relationships between continuous variables are demonstrated using correlation coefficients and linear regression. For categorical variables, the equivalent statistic is the phi coefficient. Relative risks and odds ratios are used for assessing risks and for expressing the relationship between an exposure and outcome in terms of probabilities. The concepts of number-needed-to-benefit and number-needed-to-harm help to translate relative risk into a clinically meaningful statistic.

Chapter 4

Statistical inference

Key messages

■ Inference is the process of passing from observations to generalisations. Statistically, this refers to drawing conclusions about a population from a finite number of observations made on a sample.

■ Statistical inference involves estimating a population parameter (such as mean height of schoolchildren) from a sample statistic (such as mean height in a randomly selected group of 50 children in a school) with a known degree of uncertainty.

■ Calculated from sample observations, confidence intervals provide a measure of precision of the true population value. A 95% confidence interval is thus one which, when repeatedly estimated, will 95% of the time be expected to include the true value of the parameter being estimated.

■ The formulation of a null hypothesis (the statistical hypothesis that there is no difference) is a key step in determining whether the observed differences in a study, experiment or test are true differences or simply chance findings.

■ Three factors influence the probability of rejecting the null hypothesis:
  – A large difference is less likely to arise by chance than a small one
  – A large difference is even less likely to arise by chance if the data do not vary much (low standard deviation)
  – A large difference is more likely to arise by chance with a small number of observations since even one spurious observation may have a large effect.

What is statistical inference?

Statistical inference is the process by which we extend what has been observed in a sample to say something about a wider population. If a sample is randomly drawn from a population, one might expect the characteristic of interest, for example the mean height of school-children, to differ only by some degree of random error from the true value of that characteristic in the population. Measurement of the characteristic in the sample is called a statistic, and the value of the characteristic in the population is known as a parameter. Statistical inference therefore involves estimating a population parameter from a sample statistic.

In simple random sampling, every member of the population has a known and equal probability of being included in the sample. Although this is the most desirable sampling strategy, it is common in health-related research to have samples collected using more complex designs. A practice may, for example, be interested in investigating patients' views on the introduction of an in-house relationship coun-selling service. If the views of a random sample of attendees at a GP surgery were solicited, this would probably contain few young men since they present infrequently. One solution to this problem is to increase the probability of including members of this group by modi-fying the sampling strategy to ensure that suitable quotas of young men are sampled. These more complex 'stratified' samples can still be used for statistical inference provided that appropriate adjustments are made for the systematic (non-random) errors that have been introduced. This is typically achieved by developing a model for the data that allows for the adjusting of systematic errors. It is then rea-sonable to assume that any remaining error is random, in which case statistical inference is valid and appropriate.

Estimation

The most basic case of statistical inference is point estimation, for example estimating a population mean from the mean of a sample. The sample mean will be an unbiased estimator if the expectation of the population mean from repeated sampling equals the true population mean.

The dispersion of sample means from repeated samples is a good indicator of how far our point estimate might lie from the true population mean. The standard deviation – the most widely used measure of dispersion, or variation, of a frequency distribution – summarises how widely dispersed data are around the population mean. Standard error, in contrast, refers to the standard deviation of a sample estimate; this value is used to calculate confidence intervals.

In a normal distribution, 95% of the observations lie within 1.96 standard deviations of the mean. This means that 95% of observations will fall in the range bound by the mean plus 1.96 times the standard deviation, and the mean minus 1.96 times the standard deviation. A 95% confidence interval implies that if we were to sample repeatedly, 95% of the confidence intervals would contain the true mean. So, from our single sample, we can say that we are 95% confident that the confidence interval does indeed contain the true population mean.

Confidence intervals provide a measure of precision or, expressed another way, answer the question of how good the sample (point) estimate of a population mean is. The above description has assumed that the sample mean will be normally distributed. There is a statistical rule known as the central limit theorem which shows that this assumption is almost invariably true, and this is a further reason for the normal distribution being of such central importance. The theorem goes further and states that the standard error of the statistic is directly related to the standard deviation of the data, so we do not need to take repeated data samples to obtain the standard error, one sample being sufficient.

Hypothesis-testing

Statistical inference can be used to answer questions related to experiments. Clinical trials, for example, typically compare a new treatment with an existing treatment or with a placebo. If more patients recover in the new treatment group, is this because the new intervention represents a real improvement, or is the observed difference simply a chance finding? For example, in a Tasmanian study, 753 non-asthmatic 7-year-olds had their forced expiratory volume in 1 second (FEV_1) measured. Members of the cohort were then contacted at age 30 years and asked whether they were asthmatic. Table 4.1 shows that 81/753 classified themselves as asthmatic. Those reporting asthma had an average FEV_1 of 98% predicted at age 7; the mean FEV_1 at age 7 in those not reporting asthma was slightly higher (Table 4.1). Does the observed difference indicate an association between childhood lung function and adult-onset asthma, or is this a chance finding?

We start by making the assumption that the observed difference between asthmatics and non-asthmatics occurred by chance. The probability that the observed difference did indeed arise by chance is then calculated, three factors influencing this probability:

- A large difference is *less* likely to arise by chance than a small one

- A large difference is even *less* likely to arise by chance if the data do not vary much (low standard deviation)

- A large difference is *more* likely to arise by chance with a small number of observations, since even one spurious observation may have a large effect.

If the observed difference is a chance finding, there is actually no difference; in our example, this would mean that FEV_1 at age 7 in non-asthmatic children is unrelated to an adult diagnosis of asthma.

Table 4.1 Lung function at age 7 (percentage predicted FEV_1), by adult asthmatic status

Adult asthma	n	Mean $(\bar{x})$	Standard deviation (σ)	Standard error (SE) $(\sigma/\sqrt{n})$	Confidence interval $(\bar{x}-1.96SE, \bar{x}+1.96SE)$
No	672	100.8	13.0	0.50	99.8, 101.8
Yes	81	98.0	13.5	1.5	95.1, 100.94
Difference		2.8		1.6	−0.3, 5.9

H_0 = There is no difference in lung function at age 7 by adult asthmatic status.

z = mean difference/standard error of mean difference
$$z = \frac{MD}{SE_{MD}} = \frac{2.8}{1.6} = 1.75, P = 0.08$$

This statement is called the null hypothesis, usually represented as H_0. The hypothesis that there is a difference is the alternative hypothesis, H_1. The probability we calculated is called the P value. A small P value suggests that the null hypothesis is not true and that a real difference exists. A P value of 0.05 or less is usually regarded as providing strong evidence of a true difference.

P values: uses and limitations

The P value is the probability of observing the data if the null hypothesis is true. If a difference does exist, the difference could occur in either direction; in other words, a new treatment might be either significantly better or significantly worse. To allow for either situation, we use two-sided P values. It is occasionally appropriate to use a one-sided test; if, for example, we know that a new treatment has better health outcomes and are evaluating its cost-effectiveness, we might not be interested in whether or not it is cheaper, only in whether it is significantly more expensive. One-sided tests are not commonly used, and most statistical software gives two-sided P values as the default.

P values express statistical significance, but statistically significant results may have little clinical significance. This is particularly the case with large studies that have the power to detect very small differences. For example, an improvement in average peak expiratory flow of 1 l/min seen when comparing a new asthma treatment with a placebo may be statistically significant but clearly has little clinical significance.

A further drawback of P values is the emphasis placed on P=0.05, a value chosen purely by convention but which has spawned a tendency to dismiss anything larger and focus attention on only smaller values. In contrast, the presentation of confidence intervals allows a more insightful clinical interpretation of findings.

Confidence intervals and P values

The statistical significance of differences can be gleaned from confidence intervals. A confidence interval containing 1.0 for a relative risk or an odds ratio means that we are less than 95% sure that a genuine difference exists; a significance test of the difference would thus give $P > 0.05$. Similarly, a confidence interval not including 1.0 corresponds to $P < 0.05$, whereas an interval bounded at one end by exactly 1.0 will give $P = 0.05$. A similar situation exists with confidence intervals for differences in means or proportions, the only difference being that no effect is represented by the value 0.0 rather than 1.0.

The practice of reporting both confidence intervals and P values is questionable, P values adding little information for the informed reader. An exception to this rule occurs when a large number of confidence intervals are reported; in this instance, the generally discouraged habit of replacing P values with stars indicating $P < 0.05$ and $P < 0.01$ becomes useful, allowing a rapid overview of results to be made.

Type I and type II errors

Although observed data may provide very strong evidence of an effect, the possibility of a difference arising by chance is never fully excluded. Consequently, there is always a risk that a treatment may be deemed beneficial, or an exposure harmful, when in reality it is not. Such a conclusion is known as a type I error.

Significance tests can also result in a type II error – the erroneous conclusion of no treatment benefit or no harm from exposure when the treatment is in fact beneficial or the exposure harmful. Small studies are particularly prone to type II errors; a difference may be observed, but in a small group it is hard to exclude the possibility that the difference has arisen by chance. Such studies are said to have low power to detect a difference.

Testing hypotheses between continuous variables

Testing for a difference between two means

The null hypothesis in this case is that there is no difference between two sample means. Dividing the difference between the two means by its standard error results in a statistic that can be used formally to test this hypothesis. If the value of the quotient so derived lies between

−1.96 and +1.96, there is a more than 5% probability that the observed difference is caused by chance alone, and in this case it would be unreasonable to reject the null hypothesis.

When comparing two means, one is usually the result of some observations, whereas the other might derive from previous observations or could be a hypothesised value. If the comparison is with a hypothetical value, the standard error of the sample is used in the denominator. The two sets of observations are sometimes not independent, as is the case in before and after studies in which each subject contributes a pair of observations, or when pairs of matched individuals are used. In these instances, the standard error of the difference is worked out from the differences between the paired observations.

The assumption of the normal distribution is important, and this is usually satisfied in large samples. With smaller samples, the t distribution is used in place of the normal distribution. W.S. Gossett, who wrote under the pen name 'Student', introduced the t distribution, and it is for this reason also sometimes referred to as the Student's t distribution. Like the normal distribution, the t distribution is a symmetrical, bell-shaped distribution with a mean of zero, but it is somewhat more spread out, with longer tails. Its importance lies in the fact that, in health-related research, the number of observations in experiments is often small, in which case it is appropriate to use t tests when comparing two means. In addition to the assumption of independence, t tests also assume an equal variance between groups. If variances are, however, unequal, it is necessary to use Welch's test, a discussion of which falls beyond the scope of this work.

One-way analysis of variance (ANOVA)

If we wish to compare the mean values of more than two groups, each group can be compared with all other groups by using a battery of t tests. A problem with this approach is that of 'multiple testing', this being defined most succinctly by Last as 'A problem that arises from the fact that the greater the number of statistical tests conducted on a data set, the greater is the probability that the test(s) will falsely reject the null hypothesis, solely because of the play of chance.' Thus, if, for example, we set our level of significance at 5%,

1 in 20 comparisons will be expected to be significant by chance alone. We can to some extent control for this by lowering our level of significance (to, for example, 1%) if multiple comparisons are being made.

Other techniques for adjustment also exist, perhaps the most widely used being the Bonferroni correction, in which the P value obtained is multiplied by the number of comparisons undertaken. If, for example, a P value of 0.03 were obtained in one of five comparisons made, this would be adjusted to give a P value of $0.03 \times 5 = 0.15$. For a small number of comparisons (for example, a maximum of five), its use is reasonable, but for larger numbers of comparisons it is a highly conservative approach.

If the necessity to make a multiple comparison arises from a classification of individuals on some variable (for example, nine categories of ethnicity), ANOVA can be used to test the differences between means. The null hypothesis is now that the means of all groups are equal, this being relatively straightforward to interpret if results support the null hypothesis. If, however, we obtain a P value of less than 0.05, indicating that the means are not all equal, we are left in something of a quandary since we have no idea of where the difference(s) actually lie. Positive results obtained using ANOVA will often be further investigated using descriptive statistics or a number of more complex approaches. Normality and equal variance are the main assumptions underpinning use of ANOVA.

Hypothesis-testing between categorical variables

Testing for associations

Associations between categorical variables can also be tested for statistical significance. We will consider a Bavarian study investigating the relationship between indoor heating and atopic disease in children (Box 4.1). The table shows that, in centrally heated homes, almost 8% of children suffered from hay fever, compared with just over 4% in homes heated by coal or wood. Again, we must ask whether this indicates a real association between type of heating and hay fever, the null hypothesis being that no association exists. The

Box 4.1 Example of a Chi-squared test to investigate the relationship between type of heating and hay fever

Prevalence of hay fever, by type of heating

	Hay fever (n)		
	Yes	No	*Total*
Central heating	48	569	617
Coal or wood	28	634	662
Total	76	1203	1279

The null hypothesis being tested is that there is no difference in the prevalence of hay fever between the two types of heating. For each cell, the expected value is calculated as (row total × column total) / grand total.

Expected values

	Hay fever (n)		
	Yes	No	*Total*
Central heating	$\dfrac{76\times617}{1279}=36.7$	$\dfrac{1203\times617}{1279}=580.3$	617
Coal or wood	$\dfrac{76\times662}{1279}=39.3$	$\dfrac{1203\times662}{1279}=622.7$	662
Total	76	1203	1279

The formula for a Chi-squared test is: $\chi^2 = \sum_{i=1}^{m} \dfrac{(O_i - E_i)^2}{E_i}$,

where m is equal to the number of rows (r)×the number of columns (c).

$$\chi^2 = \frac{11.3^2}{36.7} + \frac{11.3^2}{580.3} + \frac{11.3^2}{39.3} + \frac{11.3^2}{662.7} = 7.15$$

The degrees of freedom are equal to $(r-1)\times(c-1)=(2-1)\times(2-1)=1$.

For 1 degree of freedom, the critical values of Chi-squared are 3.84 for 5% significance and 6.63 for 1% significance. Our result shows that P<0.01, P actually being 0.007.

Chi-squared test allows us to differentiate between real and chance associations.

From the total numbers in each row and each column, it is possible to estimate how many children would be expected in each cell of the table if indoor heating and hay fever were unrelated, i.e. if the null hypothesis were true. The Chi-squared test does this and then compares the numbers observed with those expected. Large differences between observed and expected values suggest that the null hypothesis is not true and will result in small P values. In our example, P=0.007, indicating a 0.7% chance of the null hypothesis being true and thus providing strong evidence of an association between the type of indoor heating and hay fever. Although this test may appear very different from the significance tests for continuous data, it is based on assessing the same factors and is mathematically equivalent.

Testing for agreement

A situation in which the Chi-squared test may be incorrectly used is that of testing agreements. For example, the question of whether there is an *agreement* between two markers of medical finals exam papers is not the same as whether there is *association* between the two examiners since if one examiner always scores twice as highly as the other, there will be no agreement but a perfect association. The statistic used to test agreement is kappa, represented by κ.

If the ratings by the two raters on N subjects are cross-tabulated, the diagonal cells will contain the values for the occasions on which the raters have agreed. The sum of these frequencies divided by N will give the proportion of agreement between raters. Part of this agreement will, however, have occurred by chance. We could find the cell frequency expected as a result of chance, as in the case of a Chi-squared test, and then calculate the proportion of agreement between raters caused by chance. The maximum possible value for the proportion of agreement is 1, and if we take away the proportion of agreement caused by chance, we get the maximum possible agreement between the raters in this particular case. Similarly, the chance agreement can be removed from the observed agreement. After removing the agreement due to chance, kappa is the ratio of the proportion of agreement between raters compared with the maximum possible agreement (Box 4.2).

Another situation in which agreement is important is that between the result of a diagnostic test and the true disease state. The true disease state might be defined on the basis of a pathological test or a highly reliable diagnostic test, which is considered to be the 'gold standard'. The proportion of cases correctly diagnosed by the test is called its sensitivity, and the proportion of negative results from the tests in healthy subjects is called the specificity of the test. The proportion of correct diagnoses in positive test results is its positive predictive value, and, similarly, the proportion of healthy subjects

---

Box 4.2 Kappa test for agreement

Rater 2	Rater 1			
	a	b	c	*Total*
a	d_1			C_1
b		d_2		C_2
c			d_3	C_3
Total	R_1	R_2	R_3	T

Let two raters use a 3-point scale: a, b and c. The diagonal cells aa, bb and cc represent the situation in which they both agreed. d_i, C_i, and R_i represent the cell frequencies and marginal totals. Then, $P_o = \dfrac{\Sigma d_i}{T}$ represents the proportion of observed agreement.

When there is perfect agreement, $\Sigma d_i = T$ the ratio will be 1.

The expected frequency, e_i, for each of the diagonal cells is calculated as $\dfrac{R_i C_i}{T}$, and the proportion of agreement expected by chance is $P_e = \dfrac{\Sigma e_i}{T}$

Kappa is then calculated as $\kappa = \dfrac{P_o - P_e}{1 - P_e}$

A kappa value above 0.6 is considered to represent good agreement.

Box 4.3 Diagnostic tests

	Disease present	Disease absent	*Total*
Test positive	*a* (true positive)	*b* (false positive)	*a+b*
Test negative	*c* (false negative)	*d* (true negative)	*c+d*
Total	*a+c*	*b+d*	*n*

Sensitivity, $S=a/(a+c)$
Specificity, $Sp=d/(b+d)$
Positive predictive value, $PPV=a/(a+b)$
Negative predictive value, $NPV=d/(c+d)$
In terms of prevalence of disease (P),

$$PPV= \frac{S\times P}{(S\times P)+((1-Sp)\times(1-P))}$$

$$NPV= \frac{Sp\times(1-P)}{((1-S)\times P)+(Sp\times(1-P))}$$

Another relationship, the likelihood ratio, $LR=\dfrac{S}{1-Sp}$, is an indicator of the

certainty about a positive diagnosis after a positive test.

showing negative test results is its negative predictive value. The two predictive values are influenced by the prevalence of the disease. See Box 4.3 for more details.

Summary

Statistical inference involves estimating a population parameter from a sample statistic. The most common population parameter estimated is the population mean, this being estimated from the mean of a sample. Confidence intervals provide a measure of precision of how good the point estimate of a population mean is. Statistical inference can be used to test hypotheses in experiments. Postulating the null hypothesis is perhaps the most important step. The null hypothesis is less likely to be accepted if the effect size is large, particularly if this is observed in large, relatively homogenous samples. The probability of observing the data if the null hypothesis is true is given by the P value. Confidence intervals can also be used to present statistical significance. For continuous variables, hypothesis tests are usually used to compare the means and variances of two or more groups. In the case of categorical variables, association or agreement can be measured; distinguishing between the two is important.

Chapter 5

Study design

Key messages

■ Well-designed studies have clearly defined objectives and outcome measures.

■ Quantitative study designs can be classified into two broad categories: observational and experimental.

■ The design of a study and subsequent analysis of collected data are interconnected.

■ Incorporating a detailed plan of statistical analysis into the study protocol stage will often help in clarifying the key statistical issues that need to be considered.

■ The principal pieces of information that researchers need to make available to statisticians for calculating sample size include: the effect size that needs to be reliably detected; a measure of dispersion for continuous outcomes; the acceptable risk of error (significance and power); and predicted losses to follow-up.

So far in this book, we have concentrated on issues related to summarising data, testing associations and estimation (inference). A competent statistical analysis will not, however, rescue a study that is either poorly designed or executed. In this chapter, we consider some issues pertinent to the design of studies, focusing on the need for clear study objectives, the need to choose suitable outcome measures and the identification of an appropriate methodology to answer the question(s) being posed. The choice of study design will influence the size of the study, the data items that need to be collected and the plan of analysis.

The need for clear study objectives and outcome measures

Clear objectives

The most important aspect of designing a study is being clear about the question(s) that it is hoped the study will answer. The questions most commonly posed can be classified under three broad headings:

- *Estimating* certain population characteristics, such as the prevalence of asthma in a health authority at a particular point in time (point prevalence)

- Identifying *associations* between exposures and outcomes, such as the relationship between inhaled corticosteroid use in children and height

- Evaluating the *efficacy* and/or *effectiveness* of an intervention, such as pneumococcal vaccination in reducing incidence of pneumococcal pneumonia in adults with asthma.

These three questions sometimes follow each other in order: the scale of a problem needs to be assessed first, contributory factors are then identified, and finally potential solutions can be tested.

Clear outcome measures

Another key consideration is the choice of suitable outcome measures. Of particular importance is the need to distinguish between so-called 'primary' and 'secondary' outcome measures. Primary outcome measures are used as the basis for sample size calculations and should, ideally, satisfy certain characteristics. They should be clinically relevant, reliably measurable and comparable with those of other studies (which is increasingly important with the development of meta-analytical techniques). In a study of pneumococcal vaccination efficacy, for example, a suitable primary outcome measure might be episodes of microbiologically or serologically confirmed pneumococcal pneumonia in the 1 year period following vaccination.

It is sometimes tempting to measure surrogate outcomes; this temptation should, however, be resisted unless the surrogate measure is known to be a valid and reliable predictor of the outcome measure of interest. Considering the example of a study designed to determine the efficacy or effectiveness of pneumococcal vaccine in preventing pneumonia, a surrogate outcome that may be appropriate is serological evidence of immunity following vaccination. The difficulty with such measures lies in interpreting the clinical relevance of these findings. With very rare outcomes (for example, asthma deaths), there may be no alternative to the use of surrogate outcomes.

Choice of study design

The choice of study methodology should be determined on the basis of considerations such as the question being asked, the available resources (financial and human) and designs that reduce the risk of systematic error (bias and confounding) (Box 5.1). Study designs commonly used in health services research can be classified under two broad headings: observational and experimental studies.

Box 5.1 Sources of systematic error

- **Selection bias** refers to any error in selecting the study population such that the people who are selected to participate are not representative of the reference population, or the groups under study are not comparable

- **Information bias** refers to any error in the reporting or measurement of exposure or outcome that results in systematic differences in the accuracy of information collected between the comparison groups

- **Confounding** occurs when an estimate of the association between an exposure and an outcome is also affected by another exposure to the same disease, and the two exposures are correlated.

Observational studies

Observational studies are essentially of three types:

- Cross-sectional studies
- Cohort studies
- Case-control studies.

Cross-sectional studies provide a 'snapshot' picture at one point in time. They are therefore useful for quantifying the scale of a problem, such as the prevalence of smoking in hospitalised chronic obstructive pulmonary disease patients on a particular day of the year. Cross-sectional studies have the advantages of being relatively quick, cheap and straightforward to analyse, providing information on associations between exposure and disease (smoking and chronic obstructive pulmonary disease, for example). No information is, however, provided on causation, and it is here that cohort and case-control study designs are particularly useful.

Cohort studies follow a group over time to determine the proportion who develop the outcome of interest. Classically, these individuals will initially be disease-free, some of whom are 'exposed' and others not 'exposed' to the phenomenon of interest, the proportion who are affected in each group (for example, in terms of the development of lung cancer in smokers and non-smokers) being determined. These are sometimes referred to as prospective studies since people are identified in advance and followed up 'prospectively'. This term is, however, best avoided as it is also possible to conduct retrospective cohort studies using records that pre-date the onset of a condition and following these through time to compare disease occurrence between exposed and unexposed people.

From cohort studies, it is possible to obtain information on a temporal relationship between exposure and disease, and also to obtain an estimate of the incidence of a condition between groups, thus making it possible for a dose–response relationship to be established. The major disadvantages are that cohort studies can be slow to generate results and expensive, these problems being most acute for rare diseases, which require a large amount of observational time. The analysis of cohort studies is also often complex.

Case-control studies are better for studying rare diseases or uncommon events (such as asthma deaths), but the comparator group needs careful selection in order to avoid introducing selection bias. In these studies, people are classified on the basis of disease status. Attempts are then made to obtain an estimate of exposure to the factor(s) of interest in the two groups. Recall (information) bias is an important concern, as is the difficulty of controlling for confounding factors. Despite these reservations, case-control studies, if well conducted, offer several advantages, including quick results, efficiency and relative ease of analysis.

Experimental studies

The distinguishing feature of experimental studies is that the investigator assigns subjects to the different groups being compared; herein lies the main advantage because the risk of confounding (see Box 5.1) is greatly diminished. Randomisation confers the additional benefit of controlling for all (known and unknown) confounding factors, and it is for this reason that randomised trials represent the methodology of choice for evaluating the efficacy and effectiveness of interventions. A number of trial designs now exist, including parallel group, crossover, factorial and cluster randomised trials (Figure 5.1) A discussion of the relative strengths and weaknesses of each trial design falls beyond the scope of this chapter; those interested in pursuing this subject further are advised to refer to the further reading items detailed at the end of this book. Irrespective of the particular trial design chosen, subjects and assessors should, wherever possible, be blinded to the assigned treatment since this will, in addition, minimise the risk of information bias.

Sample size calculations

The accurate determination of sample size is a crucial aspect of study design. If the study sample is too small, a real effect may exist, and be observed, yet lack statistical significance, thus resulting in a

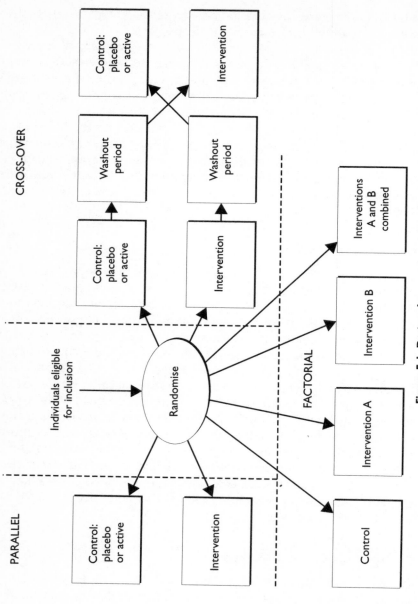

Figure 5.1 Designs for experimental studies

false-negative conclusion (also known as a type II error). On the other hand, a study that is larger than it needs to be will absorb funding that could have been better used elsewhere, and possibly delay the release of important results. Sample size calculations need to be presented in funding applications, where they are rightly subjected to close scrutiny, and they should also be clearly reported when publishing results.

Estimating sample size is complex, and for all but the simplest studies a statistician should be consulted. The questions that a statistician will ask are, however, largely predictable by those with an elementary understanding of the principles involved in calculating sample size.

Components of sample size calculations

Difference to be detected

The process of estimating the optimal number of subjects for a particular study requires researchers to think forward to the data-analysis stage. Significance tests, comparing two or more groups, seek to determine whether an observed difference is a chance finding or whether it represents a true difference between the groups. When planning the study, it is necessary to decide on the size of difference that the study will be able to detect. This should be the smallest change that is considered to be clinically important. Ideally, we want to detect any improvement, no matter how small, but because sample size increases sharply when seeking small changes, pragmatic considerations become important.

Most studies gather data on several outcomes; from these, the single most important one, commonly referred to as the 'primary outcome', should be identified. Sample size should then be based on the anticipated difference in primary outcome between the groups under study. In the case that several outcomes have equal importance, so that no primary outcome can be identified, sample size should be calculated for each outcome of interest and the largest calculated value used.

In the context of a clinical trial in which the primary outcome measure is a categorical variable, baseline disease prevalence (in the control group) needs to be known, together with the change in disease prevalence that the study seeks to detect. If the primary outcome is a continuous variable, the expected difference in the mean value is required, together with the standard deviation of the data in the control group. The required values are sometimes obtainable from the literature or from a pilot study; if this is not the case and reliable estimates are unavailable, 'best guess' clinical judgement must suffice.

Significance and power

Significance tests can result in type I or type II errors. A type I error, or false-positive, occurs when a new treatment is declared to be better than the control but is in fact no different. Conversely, concluding that the new treatment is no different when it in fact is constitutes a type II error, or false-negative result. The risk of such errors is directly related to sample size; when planning the study, it is therefore necessary to decide what risk of error is considered acceptable.

The probability of a type I error is often referred to as the significance level, typically set at 0.05 (5%). The power of a study is 1 minus the probability of a type II error. The most commonly accepted chance of a type II error is 0.2 (20%), giving a power of 0.8 (80%). In some situations, other values of significance and power will be more appropriate. If, for example, a new treatment has unpleasant side-effects, it may be appropriate to reduce the false-positive risk to 1% (0.01); for a treatment that possibly represents a major therapeutic breakthrough, the power may be increased to 90% or above.

Losses to follow-up

Participants pull out of longitudinal research studies for a number of reasons and are lost to follow-up. This usually results in exclusions from data analysis, effectively reducing the sample size. Since losses to follow-up are (almost) inevitable, it is wise to compensate at the design stage by calculating sample size normally and then multiplying up by an appropriate factor. The factor used depends on the expected losses to follow-up, best estimated from previous studies of a similar nature. In the absence of any prior knowledge, a drop-out

---

Box 5.2: Sample size calculation

Symbols used:

σ Standard deviation

ε Standard error, may be specified as a 95% confidence interval in which case

$$\varepsilon - \text{confidence interval} / 3.92$$

α Type I error rate or significance level

β Type II error rate; $1 - \beta$ refers to the power

$z_{2\alpha}$ Standardised normal deviate of two-tailed probability of α

$z_{2\beta}$ Standardised normal deviate of two-tailed probability of β

π Proportion

n Sample size

d Difference between means

Numerical subscripts will be used to show different groups.

Sample size for mean of a single sample:

Information required: standard deviation, standard error

Formula: $n > \dfrac{\sigma^2}{\varepsilon^2}$

Example: If, in a population, the standard deviation of serum albumin is 5.84 g/l, how large a sample is required to estimate mean serum albumin level with a confidence interval of 1 g/l?

$\sigma = 5.84 \, \text{g/l}$

$\varepsilon = 1/3.92 = 0.255 \, \text{g/l}$

$n >= \dfrac{\sigma^2}{\varepsilon^2} = \dfrac{5.84^2}{0.255^2} = 524.5 = 525$ individuals.

Sample size for proportion of a single sample:

Information required: proportion, standard error

Formula: $n > \dfrac{\pi (1 - \pi)}{\varepsilon^2}$

Box 5.2: Sample size calculation (*continued*)

Example: If one.in four schoolchildren experiences wheeze in the previous 12 months, how many schoolchildren should be included in a survey to determine the proportion of children with wheeze with a standard error of 2%?

$$n > \frac{\pi(1-\pi)}{\varepsilon^2} = \frac{0.25 \times 0.75}{0.0004} = 468.75 \text{ or } 469 \text{ children.}$$

Sample size for difference between two means:

Information required: standard deviation, difference between means, significance level, power

Formula: $n > 2\left[\dfrac{(z_{2\alpha}+z_{2\beta})\sigma}{d}\right]^2$

Example: A randomised-controlled trial is to be carried out to compare the efficacy of a new bronchodilator with salbutamol in patients with established asthma. The primary outcome is morning peak expiratory flow, a difference of greater than 5% being considered to be clinically important. The trial is required to have 80% power at the 5% significance level. From the literature, it is estimated that adult asthmatics have an average morning peak expiratory flow rate of 400l/min, with a standard deviation of 100l/min. 20 l/min (5% of 400 l/min) will be the clinically significant difference.

$$n > 2\left[\frac{(z_{2\alpha}+z_{2\beta})\sigma}{d}\right]^2 = 2\left[\frac{(1.96+0.842)\times100}{20}\right]^2 = 392.56 = 393 \text{ individuals}$$

---

rate of 20% may be assumed. If the sample size is then increased by 25%, it will be returned to the original value by a 20% drop-out rate.

Unequal groups

The most statistically efficient study design will always have equally sized groups, although other considerations sometimes still make an unbalanced study the best option. If a case-control design is used to study a rare disease, the number of available cases may be limited, or if a new treatment is particularly expensive, it may be cost-effective, for example, to compare a small number of treated patients with a larger number who are untreated. To compensate for the lower efficiency of an unbalanced design, the overall sample size needs to increase – reducing the number of patients in one arm of a trial thus requires an increase of greater magnitude in the other arm. As the design moves further from a 1:1 ratio, to 2:1, 3:1 or 4:1, greater compensation is required. The statistical inefficiency of unbalanced studies should therefore be weighed against the practical considerations militating against a balanced study design.

Box 5.2 gives formulae and examples of sample size calculations.

Summary

Statisticians are unable to salvage poorly designed or executed studies. Clearly defined study objectives and outcomes measures, and appropriate attention to sample size calculations, are some of the key features of well-designed studies. Quantitative studies can conveniently be classified into observational and experimental study designs.

Chapter 6

Combining studies: systematic reviews and meta-analyses

Key messages

■ Systematic reviews of the literature are now regarded as the gold standard approach to investigating the effectiveness of healthcare interventions.

■ Transparency is the hallmark of well-conducted systematic reviews. They are characterised by a focused research question (which is typically clinical in nature), a comprehensive search strategy for both published and unpublished data, uniformly applied selection criteria for the inclusion of studies, and the rigorous critical appraisal and summarising of data.

■ Systematic reviews should be treated as any other piece of original research, with work proceeding in a methodological manner according to an agreed protocol.

■ A quantitative synthesis of data from separate but similar studies is known as a meta-analysis. This pooling of information increases the precision of estimates of effectiveness (or other outcomes of interest) and also increases the external validity of findings when compared with individual studies.

■ Meta-analysis is not always clinically and/or statistically appropriate, in which case data can be qualitatively synthesised.

Why do we need systematic literature reviews?

In previous chapters, we focused on results obtained from single research studies. Single studies are, however, typically insufficient in themselves to unequivocally answer research questions on a particular question. It is thus commonplace to find a number of studies on a given question. In view of the sheer volume of research evidence now accumulated and the speed with which it is being generated, it is now increasingly difficult for health professionals to keep abreast of all developments in their own fields of interest, let alone the whole of medicine. Review articles have emerged as an important and essential tool for summarising knowledge in a given area. Reviews themselves are, however, subject to systematic and random errors, and the notion of systematic reviews has emerged in an attempt to reduce such errors. A detailed appreciation of the steps involved in conducting systematic reviews should help readers of these reviews to be in a position to assess their quality.

Steps in conducting a systematic review

Define the research question

The first and most crucial step in conducting a systematic review is to define the research question clearly. Unlike many narrative reviews, systematic reviews typically address a very focused question. The main advantage of taking time to crystallise the question is that this will make the rest of the task easier, and the process is thus much more likely to yield easily interpretable results. Trying to address every aspect of a problem will in contrast result in answers that are at best difficult to interpret and at worst meaningless. If the range of issues to which one is seeking answers is broad, it is good practice to identify several focused questions and undertake separate systematic reviews for each.

The following questions may help in focusing the research question:

- What is the problem to be studied?

- In which population is the problem to be studied?

- What is the intervention to be studied?

- What is the intervention being compared with?
- What is the primary outcome measure of interest?
- What are the secondary outcomes?
- Which study designs are to be included?

Once the research question has been finalised, the next step is to prepare the review protocol. This is an important and *sine qua non* step for a systematic review. Systematic reviews are planned investigations, and, as with any other research, the plan should be finalised before proceeding with the main research.

Preparing the protocol

Preparation of the protocol forces reviewers to consider the entire review process and should help to identify potential problems at an early stage. It is good practice to have the methods to be used independently scrutinised at this stage. As an agreed document, it serves as a reference throughout the review process and can be published, thereby minimising the tendency on the part of some researchers to make *post hoc* changes to the research question. An example of a systematic review protocol is given in Box 6.1. The protocol may also include a timetable for the review and a budget.

Scoping search

Before proceeding with the systematic review, it is important to ensure that there are no reviews with the same focus either existing or in progress. A scoping search of major electronic databases such as the Cochrane Library, Medline, Embase and the National Research Register should help to identify other systematic reviews on the same or similar questions. The scoping search and protocol development often proceed concurrently.

Conducting detailed searches: where to search

The validity and usefulness of a systematic review depend at least in part on the comprehensiveness of the searches that have been

Box 6.1   Example of a systematic review protocol demonstrating key features

This example demonstrates some of the salient features of a review protocol. For a fuller description of the protocol, please refer to: Alves B, Sheikh A, Hurwitz B, Durham SR. Allergen injection immunotherapy for seasonal allergic rhinitis (Protocol for a Cochrane Review). In: *The Cochrane Library*, Issue 2, 2003. Oxford: Update Software.

Title
Allergen injection immunotherapy for seasonal allergic rhinitis.

Objectives
To evaluate the benefit and harm of injection immunotherapy in the management of people suffering from seasonal allergic rhinitis.

Criteria for considering studies for this review
Types of study
Randomised, double-blind, placebo-controlled trials.
Types of participant
Patients with seasonal allergic rhinitis caused by tree, grass or weed pollens. Allergy must be proven using objective tests of allergy such as skin prick tests or the radioallergoabsorbent test (RAST).
Types of intervention
Multiple injections of high-dose immunotherapy with standardised single allergen extracts compared with placebo.
Main outcome measures
Improvements in symptoms and disease-specific quality of life.

Search strategy for the identification of studies
Searches of Medline, Embase and the Cochrane Trials Register. Contacting the first-named authors of identified studies to locate additional unpublished data.

Methods of review
Two independent reviewers will check titles and abstracts identified from the searches. Both reviewers will obtain the full text of all studies of possible relevance for assessment. The reviewers will decide which trials fit the inclusion criteria and grade their methodological quality. Any disagreement will be resolved by discussion between the reviewers. Authors will be contacted for clarification where necessary.

undertaken. Searches are typically undertaken of the major biomedical electronic databases, specialist databases, the so-called 'grey' literature (books, theses and reports) and the Internet. In addition, research centres and individuals with known expertise in the area should be contacted in an attempt to locate unpublished literature. Searching the bibliographies of key publications can help to identify additional literature that is potentially of relevance. Details of some of the more useful electronic data sources to consider searching are detailed in Box 6.2.

Conducting detailed searches: search terms

Having large electronic databases of studies is only useful if the relevant studies can easily and efficiently be identified. Considerable effort has been expended in recent years in developing detailed search strategies. Most electronic databases keep records with tagged fields, and all records are also indexed using medical subheadings (MeSH). Building a search strategy involves selecting the fields to be searched and choosing the relevant MeSH terms. Wildcards ($) can also be used so that only a part of the word is specified; thus 'rand$' will simultaneously search for words such as 'randomised', 'randomized', 'randomisation', 'randomization', etc.

One may specify how two or more words occur, either as an exact phrase or together within some specified block of text. Boolean operators such as 'AND', 'OR' and 'NOT' can also be used to combine different searches. Search strategies can be tested against a gold standard to define their specificity and sensitivity. These gold standards are usually defined by hand-searching a core group of journals spanning a specified period. A search is said to be highly specific if the results exclude irrelevant records. It is termed highly sensitive if it includes most relevant records. As can be expected, a trade-off between sensitivity and specificity of searches exists in practice.

Search strategies usually include at least three dominant concepts or fields: searches on the subject of interest, the intervention of interest and study type(s). For example, if we are interested in assessing the effectiveness of immunotherapy in the treatment of people with hay fever, we would devise searches around each of

Box 6.2 Some sources of studies for systematic reviews

Cochrane Central Register of Controlled Trials (CENTRAL)
A regularly updated bibliography of publications that report on controlled trials. Available from: www.nelh.nhs.uk

Cumulative Index to Nursing and Allied Health Literature (CINAHL)
Includes titles from over 1200 journals and more than half a million records plus abstracts and selected full text from 1982 onwards. Available from: www.cinahl.com/cdirect/cdirect.htm

Database of Abstracts of Reviews of Effectiveness (DARE)
Contains abstracts of systematic reviews and references to other reviews, which may be useful for background information. Available from: www.york.ac.uk/inst/crd/revs.htm

Excerpta Medica database (EMBASE)
Covers 4000 pharmaceutical and biomedical journals from 1974 onwards. Available from: www.embase.com

LILACS
A database of more than 600 regional journals from Latin America and the Caribbean. Available from: www.unifesp.br/suplem/cochrane/lilacs.htm

MEDLINE (PUBMED)
Covers more than 4600 journals and over 11 million abstracts from 1966 onwards. This now also incorporates the Healthstar database. Available from: www.pubmed.gov

NLMGateway
In addition to Medline, the NLM Gateway searches LOCATORplus, MEDLINEplus, ClinicalTrials.gov, DIRLINE, AIDS Meetings, Health Services Research Meetings, Space Life Sciences Meetings, and HSRProj databases. Available from: http://gateway.nlm.nih.gov

Psychological Abstracts (PsycINFO)
Has about two million abstracts and citations to literature in behavioural sciences and mental health from 1800 journals, books, chapters from books and dissertations. Available from: www.apa.org/psychinfo

Zetoc
An electronic table of contents service from the British Library. The database includes 19 million journal and conference records from some 20000 journals. Available from: zetoc.mimas.ac.uk

the three main fields of interest: hay fever, immunotherapy and randomised controlled studies (as these represent the study design of choice for evaluating the effectiveness of treatments).

Biases in searching: problems of publication bias and duplicate publications

There are many limitations to searches of electronic databases that need to be considered when devising the detailed search strategy. They do not, for example, cover all published journals, and they have a bias towards English language publications. Among the journals covered, not all papers are recorded, this being a problem that is particularly relevant to the indexing of older papers. More seriously, not all conducted studies are published, this being a particular problem in relation to studies that fail to find significant outcomes. The tendency to submit and publish papers based on the direction and strength of their effect is known as publication bias. Therefore, for a systematic review to be comprehensive, it has actively to pursue and find studies. Unpublished studies can be traced from hand-searching key journals, conference abstracts, dissertations and theses, reports, White Papers, funding sources and the Internet. The authors of papers should always be contacted as they have the greatest familiarity with research in their fields. Departments and institutes with research in the field of interest might also have such unpublished studies.

A contrasting concern is the problem posed by duplicate publications, this referring to the biases introduced through repeated publications of the same data. This is a particular problem in relation to studies showing positive benefits associated with the introduction of new treatments. Such studies therefore need to be identified and treated as a single study. A list of reporting biases is given in Box 6.3.

Selecting studies

Detailed in the review protocol should be clear inclusion and exclusion criteria in a form that can be applied to the search results without ambiguity. Shifting inclusion/exclusion criteria during the review process is a potentially important source of bias. To further minimise the risk of such bias, all decisions about whether or not to

---

Box 6.3 Publication bias and other reporting biases

Publication bias – The publication or non-publication of research findings, depending on the nature and direction of the results. Since the bias is towards publishing significant results, a method of finding publication bias is to show that studies with a small sample size will, if published, have a large effect size. A graphical way of presenting this is by using the funnel plot. When the effect sizes from different trials are plotted against a measure of their precision such as sample size or inverse of the standard error, trials with lower precision will have wider variations in their effect size. As precision increases, variation narrows, giving the graph an inverted funnel appearance. If the direction and strength of effect do not influence publication, the 'funnel' will be symmetrical, but in the presence of publication bias it will be asymmetrical.

Time lag bias – The delayed or rapid publication of research findings depending on the nature and direction of the results. Trials with negative results are often published after a longer delay than those with positive results.

Multiple publication bias – The multiple or singular publication of research findings, depending on the nature and direction of the results.

Citation bias – The citation or non-citation of research findings depending on the nature and direction of the results.

Language bias – Publishing in certain languages depending on the nature and direction of the results. Positive findings tend to be published in international English journals, whereas negative findings are published in local languages.

Outcome reporting bias – The selective reporting of some outcomes and not others depending on the nature and direction of the results.

---

include studies should be made by at least two people working independently with clearly defined processes for handling any disagreements that may arise; this usually involves a third person who can act as an arbitrator between co-reviewers.

The process of selecting studies typically proceeds in a phased manner. As searches are usually maximally sensitive, many reports that are not relevant to the review question will be identified. A preliminary title and abstract screen allows the identification of potentially useful studies, and full papers of these studies should be obtained. Full papers will then again be assessed against the predefined inclusion criteria and a quality assessment process (see below); studies satisfying these criteria will be included in the review. The majority of studies identified will typically have been excluded, and it is good practice to keep a log of which studies have been excluded, together with a record of the reasons for exclusion. Many journals now require this information to be explicitly presented in a flow diagram as part of a 'quality of reporting of meta-analyses' (QUOROM) statement. An example of a flow diagram is given in Box 6.4.

Assessing the quality of selected studies

Quality is difficult to assess reliably so this step is therefore sometimes somewhat subjective. A detailed discussion of the methods for assessing study quality is not possible within the confines of this book, but suffice it to say that quality assessment depends largely on an assessment of internal validity and, to a lesser extent, external validity. Internal validity refers to the extent to which results from a study can be believed, that is, specific efforts have been made to exclude the impact of chance, bias and confounding contributing to the observed results. There are many checklists and scales for quality assessment; in essence, these focus on assessing issues such as concealment of allocation, blinding and completeness of follow-up data.

The major influences on the quality of a study come from the factors that determine internal validity. The results of a given study will be correct only if adequate precautions have been taken to prevent systematic error in allocating subjects to the different groups, the groups receive similar care except for the intervention of interest, outcomes are measured similarly in all groups, and loss to follow-up is similar in all groups. External validity refers to how generalisable the results are. There is no consensus on what to do with quality scores. A reasonable use will be in sensitivity analysis to test how the quality of the trial has affected its result. Quality scores might be used to weight the study results when they are pooled, or pooling may be done cumulatively, studies being ranked according to quality.

Box 6.4 A QUOROM flow chart of the process of identifying and selecting studies

This example is from a systematic review investigating ethnic variations in asthma prevalence, morbidity and health services utilisation. Studies were included if they contained UK data on asthma prevalence, morbidity or health service utilisation in at least one minority ethnic group and in indigenous Whites and conducted between 1981 and 2001.

Searches yielded 2086 non-duplicate papers from nine electronic databases; one study was identified through cross-reference; one, an unpublished dissertation, was pointed out by an expert contacted; another study was identified through searching the Internet. The search results were screened to identify potentially relevant studies.

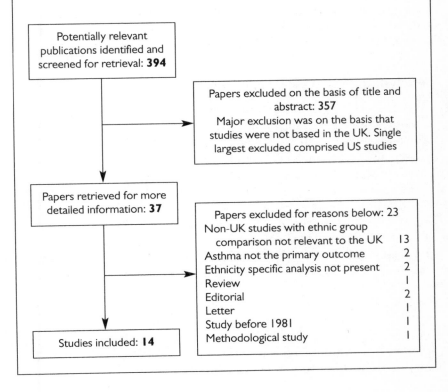

Data extraction

Data from individual studies are collected onto a piloted data extraction form. The data extraction form will have fields to show the identity of the reviewer and the date, and key identifying details for the study, including the study title, first author and source and date of publication. Data extraction forms should allow the easy extraction of information on parameters such as the location of the study, its time frame, a description of the participants with relevant age, sex and other demographic details, the number of study groups, interventions, placebo, details of assessing the quality of methods, the number of participants in each group at the beginning and at every point of measurement and, importantly, details of the results. Piloting the form on a few study reports often helps to improve its usefulness. Two reviewers should independently extract data, and, in an attempt to further minimise risk of bias, reviewers may be blinded to the study authors, institutions and journals. This is especially useful if a quality score is going to be integrated into the analysis.

Analysis and interpretation of results

The results of a systematic review should contain details of the studies that are included and those that are excluded, together with the reasons for exclusion. This helps readers to assess the findings of the review. This and the explicitly stated methodology are two of the main differences between a traditional and a systematic review. The characteristics of the studies included should be presented in a table. Binary outcome measures are usually calculated as odds ratios or relative risks. Continuous measures are expressed as the difference between means or in their standardised form. The study results can be graphically presented as a Forrest plot. In this representation, each study is represented by a black square, the area of which can be varied to represent the weight of the study when pooling results. A horizontal line passing through the square represents the 95% confidence interval. A vertical line is sometimes placed to indicate no effect. Figure 6.1 is an example of a meta-analysis of eight studies demonstrating differences in the diagnosis of clinician-diagnosed asthma in White and South Asian children.

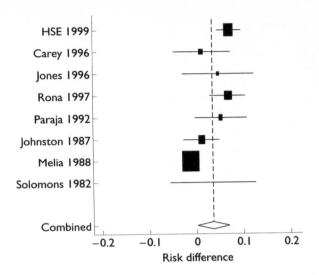

Figure 6.1 Meta-analysis of eight studies showing risk difference in clinician-diagnosed asthma between Whites and South Asians

It is not necessary to combine studies to produce a single value for effect size. The study results can be discussed, and a qualitatively synthesised conclusion can be reached. If the study results are combined, that process of pooling is called meta-analysis. The methods of meta-analysis are described in the next section.

Meta-analysis

Combining results from different studies to produce an overall quantitative summary measure of treatment effect is called meta-analysis. When conducted appropriately, this offers the advantage of increasing the precision of an estimate and, furthermore, by drawing on the results of studies conducted in different settings and locations, enhances the generalisability of the conclusions reached. But pooling of data is not always the right thing to do and can, if performed inappropriately, result in erroneous conclusions.

Is pooling appropriate?

The first question to be asked when contemplating whether or not to pool data relates to whether this is clinically appropriate. Thus, although pooling data from trials of antibiotic use in children with tonsillitis is likely to be clinically appropriate, pooling the results of studies evaluating the effectiveness of antibiotics for tonsillitis in otherwise healthy and immunocompromised children might not be as appropriate. This is above all a clinical judgement, and the views of (a number of) clinicians should be sought if there is any doubt.

If studies are considered to be clinically homogenous, the next question to ask is whether they are statistically homogenous enough to consider pooling. There are two broad schools of thought here: the first arguing that statistically heterogeneous studies should not be pooled, the other making the case for the careful pooling of such data using random effects models and investigating where the heterogeneity lies through stratified subgroup analyses (discussed in more detail below).

Calculating summary statistics for individual studies

If it is felt clinically appropriate to pool data from different studies, a key first step in meta-analysis is to calculate summary statistics for each study. The summary statistics calculated depend on the type of outcome variable. In the case of binary outcome variables, odds ratios, relative risks and risk differences are the most frequently used measures of effect. In the case of continuous variables, a key question is whether studies have used the same or different scales to measure the outcome of interest. If the same scale has been used, the difference between means can be used, but if different scales have been used, the summary statistics will need to be expressed in a standardised form (i.e. a standardised difference in means will be used).

Pooling of data from individual studies

The second main step in meta-analysis is the actual pooling of the summary statistics. One issue to be resolved here is to decide whether the studies included are sufficiently similar to one another (or homogenous) to render the process valid. If the studies are very different, pooling their results will not yield valid interpretable results, and a meta-analysis should not be undertaken. At the other extreme, when studies show little variability, one can assume that the studies are all measuring a true or 'fixed' effect and that the differences observed between studies are due to chance alone. This is called the fixed effects model meta-analysis.

Between these two cases lies the random effects model. In this model, the underlying concept is that the true value does not have a single fixed value but instead follows some probability distribution. The expected variability is therefore greater than would be seen with fixed effects, but it is still considered reasonable to combine studies and calculate an overall effect. If a study characteristic contributing to heterogeneity is known, studies can be stratified on that characteristic and analysed.

Other methods for pooling data exist, but these are less commonly used than the fixed and random effects models techniques described above. For binary outcomes, for example, Mantel–Haenszel methods are more suitable when the data are sparse. Peto's odds ratio method is claimed to be assumption-free and hence can be used in situations where either fixed or random effects models are considered appropriate.

Summary

Systematic reviews attempt to reduce the risk of bias inherent in traditional reviews in order to allow valid and reliable summaries of the literature to be obtained. Reviews should seek to answer a clearly stated and focused research question. Well-conducted systematic reviews are undertaken in accordance with an *a priori* agreed review protocol that has been subjected to independent peer review. Searches should be comprehensive, seeking to identify the relevant published and unpublished data; the latter are particularly important to locate in order to minimise the risk of publication bias. Explicitly stated criteria are used to select relevant, high-quality studies for inclusion. Statistical pooling of results from different studies may be appropriate, this judgement depending on both clinical and statistical considerations.

Chapter 7

Managing data

Key messages

- Data collection and processing are important steps that need to be considered in detail before embarking on a research project.

- The careful selection of an appropriate statistical package will pay dividends in the long run.

- It is now relatively easy to transfer data between spreadsheets and statistical packages.

- Keeping a detailed log of the various steps undertaken during data analysis is important to allow replication of the results at a future point.

Developing efficient mechanisms for the collection and processing of data is an important step and one that that needs to be considered at the protocol design stage by those undertaking research projects. Even after completing the research, there is the need to ensure safe storage of the data. This is so that detailed and accurate records can be accessed in order to undertake any secondary analyses of data that may in the future be deemed important or, more fundamentally, to furnish evidence, should it be required, that the research in question actually took place.

In this final chapter, we discuss some of the practicalities of data collection and then describe the steps needed in order to transform data that have been collected into a form that is suitable for analysis. We consider issues of how best to organise the data, the usefulness of database software and the choice of statistical software. Also mentioned are a number of practical tips that we hope will ease the process of data management, since the tasks involved need not be onerous.

Data collection

Data collection can be expensive in terms of time and money. A key point to remember is that collecting a large number of poor quality data is seldom helpful for answering either the main question or indeed questions that may subsequently arise. The temptation simply to collect 'as much data as possible' on the grounds that a similar opportunity might not again arise should therefore be resisted by all except the most experienced researchers. The main problem with such a blanket approach to data collection is that data quality might suffer, thereby jeopardising the ability of the study to yield meaningful answers.

All data should be identifiable in terms of who collected them, and where and when this occurred. It is not unknown for records to be misplaced, forgotten or, in our current electronic age, wiped out. To minimise the risks of such potentially fatal errors, paper records should be copied and safely stored, and data in electronic form should be regularly backed up.

Organising data

Data are usually arranged in a grid, each row representing an individual and each column a variable. It is seldom necessary to identify individuals retrospectively, so names and addresses need not be entered because, if present, these constitute an unnecessary confidentiality risk. Instead, a unique identifier should be used in files containing data, and a list mapping identifiers to individuals should be stored securely elsewhere.

The unique identifier may simply be the row number, or it may contain more information. For example, in a study in which several general practices contribute up to 100 patients each, a three-digit number might be used, the first digit indicating the practice and the next two digits a patient from that practice. For larger studies, data are more manageable if stored in a number of smaller files instead of one large one. The unique identifier can then be used to link the different files together. Statistical packages readily merge data from separate files, although the records in each file usually need to be sorted in order of the identifier.

Data entry

Data can be entered either using a database package or directly into a statistical package. For larger studies, the use of a dedicated database package such as Microsoft Access is advisable, although data then need to be transferred to a statistical package for analysis. One advantage of using database software is a reduced number of errors since erasing or altering data is made deliberately difficult. For smaller studies, data may be entered directly into the statistics package. Before entering any values, the variables should be defined, this definition telling the computer what to expect and further reducing the chance of error. In Access, this is done in the 'design view' window, and in the Statistical Packages for Social Scientists (SPSS), it is most easily achieved by right-clicking at the top of a column and choosing 'define variable'.

Before data are entered, a number of important decisions may need to be taken. One very common consideration concerns the way in which categorical variables will be coded. Most statistical packages require categorical variables to be numerically coded before they are used in analyses. Numerical data should be entered with the same precision as they were noted. The formatting of date and time should be consistent. If data from the same individual are entered into different datasets, there should be a variable to link records between different databases.

Defining variables

Each variable in a dataset is defined by name, type and format. The variable name should ideally be sufficiently descriptive to facilitate easy recognition of the category of data being entered. Depending on the statistical application being used, there might be restrictions on the type and number of characters a variable name can have. Although long descriptive variable names are useful, there is often a trade-off that needs to be considered since a number of such variables might need to be entered into a statistical command. The concern here is that some statistical applications have a limit to the number of characters that can be used in any one command.

Questionnaire information falls into two main categories: numeric and textual (string). Although either type of data may be entered onto a computer, numeric variables allow easier analysis and a more reliable transfer between packages. Textual data should therefore, wherever possible, be coded numerically; for example, the frequency of asthma exacerbations being reported as daily/weekly/monthly/annually could be coded as 1/2/3/4.

Labels

Variable labels are a short description of what the variable is. They are especially useful if variable names are not descriptive. Similarly, labels for values in numerically coded categorical variables can also be assigned. It is good practice to ensure that all variables and values have labels; most statistical packages now display these labels and may use them in their outputs.

Data-checking

Data should routinely be checked for errors. The types of error that can occur during data entry are too numerous to list but range from a simple transposition of digits to missing decimal points to the more serious problem of missing fields and even, in some cases, entire records. A common error is the lack of uniqueness of fields where this would otherwise be expected – unique patient records are an obvious example of a data field for which one would not anticipate finding more than one entry.

Small amounts of data can be manually checked. With larger amounts, it is important that measures for controlling data errors are considered from the outset of the study. The training of data entry personnel is crucial in this respect, and in practice this is often done during a run-in period using mock datasets before actual study data entry takes place. Once consistency and reliability have been achieved, batch sampling can be used to check the quality of data entry. Errors can be reduced by independent double entry of the data, with agreement over what to do in the event of discrepancy. Data entry programs allow logical checks to be run as data are entered. An example of such a check is to ascertain whether the data entered fall within a prespecified range (for example, 0–100 for age). After data entry has been completed, running frequencies and other descriptive statistics may also discover errors.

In most cases, it is possible, once they have been identified, to correct errors that may have crept in during data entry. If for any reason, however, these errors cannot be corrected, it is often necessary to discard the relevant part of the data field.

Missing data

Missing data can cause problems when transferring data between packages. This is often particularly problematic if the number of items in each row of the database varies since values may be read into the wrong column and may remain undetected. The easiest way to prevent this problem is to enter something into every box, using an implausible value where data are missing. If, for example, age is missing, enter '999'. The computer must then know not to include these values. In SPSS, the missing value can be included in the definition; in packages without this facility, the value should be recoded as missing immediately before analysis.

Data may be missing for a number of reasons, such as incomplete filling-in of questionnaires or incomplete recording of the findings. There are a number of approaches to handling such missing data during analyses. The most common approach is to assume that data are missing at random, but this assumption should be verified. When data are missing at random, removing the records with incomplete data should not affect the validity of the findings. This does, however, lead to a reduction in sample size; if this is not accounted for in the original sample size calculations, it can lead to a loss of statistical power. Another approach is to replace missing values by a group mean or other such value. In the case of longitudinal studies, the last value of a variable can be used to replace the missing value. Most statistical packages have some method for inputting missing data, but it should be remembered that the default is often case-wise or list-wise deletion. A problem with deletion is that analyses involving different variables might be carried out using different base samples.

Choosing a statistical package

Two statistical packages are widely used in medical research: SPSS and Stata. SPSS tends to be favoured by the less statistically adept because it is relatively easy to use, the type of analysis to be undertaken usually being selected from a drop-down menu. Stata is, in contrast, command driven and therefore requires the user to learn at least the basic set of commands. For anyone planning to do a significant number of analyses, however, the effort of learning Stata will pay dividends in the longer term. Once the basics have been mastered, Stata is straightforward to use and gives a feeling of being in control, whereas SPSS feels, in contrast, more of a 'black box' approach. Alternatives to SPSS and Stata include Epi-Info, a basic package available free from the Internet, and SAS, which is very difficult to use but is one of the few programs available that are capable of handling extremely large datasets. Stata has a special edition (Stata/SE), which can also handle large datasets.

The statistical tests described in this book are in reality quite simple, and most can be carried out using a general-purpose spreadsheet program such as Microsoft Excel, which has a good built-in data analysis module. For more advanced analyses, Excel statistical 'add-ins' are also available, which increase the range of statistical tests that can be performed. The main advantages of Excel are its widespread availability and ease of use.

When choosing which statistical application to work with, one would do well to consider the following four questions:

- Does the particular application have the facility to perform the analyses I want to undertake? Certain analyses are often more easily or better executed in certain applications

- Are the data available in a form that is acceptable to the application? Before data can be transported between applications, they may need to be translated, which in itself may require specialist data-translation software

- Is the application supported by the operating system of my computer?

- Are there any limitations inherent in the application? This is particularly important in the case of free downloads and trial software. Vital functions such as 'save' are sometimes disabled in these, and others will use only a proportion of the data entered for analysis.

Transferring data between packages

Data transfer is much easier than it used to be, and it is now frequently possible to save data from one package directly into the format of another. If this is not possible, a good intermediate format is the 'comma-separated variables' (csv) file, which can be created and read by most commercially available packages.

It is, however, still easy for data to become corrupted during transfer because of missing values. The problem of blank fields has already been described. A further problem is that the definition of a missing value might be lost so a value such as 999 may be erroneously included in the analysis. A good check on the data, once they have been transferred, is to calculate a few summary statistics such as mean age, age range or the proportion of males and compare these results with those obtained using the original package; this simple process will usually bring to light whether anything has gone wrong during data transfer.

Repeatable results

It is good practice to be able to recreate the results of an analysis, enabling the work to be readily checked if necessary. SPSS is usually run interactively by clicking on the drop-down menus and windows, but in our experience it is often hard to go back and remember exactly what was done. The answer is to use the syntax window, in which the actual commands used by SPSS are visible. To use this facility, select an analysis in the usual way but before clicking 'OK', click 'Paste'; the syntax then appears in a separate window and can be saved in a file. On returning to the analysis, this file can be opened and run to repeat the analysis exactly. With a little experience, it is possible to learn to modify these commands if necessary.

Being able to repeat analyses in Stata is easier. The commands used simply need to be stored in a text file with a '.do' extension. On returning to Stata, the command 'do filename' will re-run the commands as before; to make changes, the file can be edited and then re-run. Statistical analysis of the data is frequently an iterative process, small changes being made after discussion with colleagues; such changes are much easier when analyses are programmed to be repeatable.

Data are often changed during the course of analysis. Some variables may be recoded or transformed into new variables, and some records may need to be dropped from certain analyses. It is important to maintain a record of all such changes. In the case of a secondary analysis of the existing data, all modifications should be clearly mentioned in the published report so that someone else can replicate the process used and obtain the same results.

Summary

Efficient data collection and management are important and integral components of successful research endeavours. When designing a study, careful consideration should be given to the data items that are to be collected. Once collected, data should be carefully organised, with agreed mechanisms for minimising errors during data entry and protecting confidentiality. There are a number of statistical packages commercially available; time taken in choosing an appropriate statistical package will, in the long run, pay important dividends.

Glossary

This glossary aims to give succinct and, we hope, user-friendly definitions of some of the more important statistical terms introduced in this book. We hope that these will also serve as an *aide-memoire* to some of the statistical concepts discussed in the preceding pages. Those interested in more detailed statistical definitions and details of statistical tests and their derivations are advised to consult a statistical or epidemiological dictionary.

agreement When the results of two measurements yield the same value for an outcome, the two measurements are said to be in agreement; the extent of this agreement can be assessed using a kappa score.

alternative hypothesis The hypothesis that a treatment is effective or groups are different; this therefore stands in contradistinction to the null hypothesis, which postulates that there is no difference between groups.

association Statistical dependency between two or more variables. Correlation (see below) is a special case of association.

bias Systematic deviation from the truth.

case-control study Cases who have an identified outcome of interest (typically a disease state) are identified, and their past exposure to suspected aetiological risk factors is compared with that of controls who do not have the outcome of interest.

coefficient of variation Standard deviation relative to the mean. This is calculated as the ratio of standard deviation to the mean and usually expressed as a percentage.

cohort A group sharing a common characteristic.

cohort study A cohort (see above) is followed through time to determine the proportion who develop an outcome of interest. These will classically be disease-free individuals, one group who are 'exposed', another group not 'exposed' to possible risk factor(s). The proportion of each group who are affected is then determined.

confidence interval A range constructed around the sample statistic in such a way that the population parameter is included with a specified probability.

confidence level The probability that the confidence interval will include the parameter.

confounding Distortion of an association by other factors that influence both the exposure and the outcome under study.

correlation A linear association between two variables.

data Factual information used for making inferences or predictions.

dependent variable Outcome variable.

distribution The spread of a variable within a sample or population.

effect size The standardised difference between the means of experimental and control groups.

epidemiology The study of the distribution of health and disease in specified populations in order to understand their causes and the burden they pose.

error The difference of a measured value from the true value. Errors may result from either chance (random error) or bias (systematic error).

estimation A rule by which a population parameter is derived from a sample statistic.

external validity An assessment of the generalisability of study results.

fixed effects model meta-analysis An approach to the statistical pooling of studies in which it is assumed that all studies are measuring a true or 'fixed' effect and that differences between studies are thus the result simply of chance.

hypothesis A theory, resulting from reflection or observation, that can be tested and refuted.

incidence The rate at which new cases occur in a population during a specified period.

independent variable An explanatory or predictor variable.

intercept The point at which the regression line crosses the y-axis.

internal validity The extent to which it is possible, after taking account of study methods, to conclude that the relationship observed in a study may, apart from sampling error, be attributed to the hypothesised effect under investigation.

kurtosis The extent to which data with a unimodal distribution are peaked.

mean Arithmetic mean (or average) is calculated by summing all the observations and then dividing the sum by the number of observations.

measurement Measurement involves mapping an aspect of an object onto a measurement scale according to some specified rules.

measurement scales, types There are four types of scale:

Nominal – labels or names that identify persons or objects according to some characteristic

Ordinal – when categories in a nominal scale can be ranked and ordered

Interval – in addition to classifying and ordering, an interval scale allows us to make inferences about the differences between categories. If the numerical difference between two points in a pair of points is equal to the same difference between another pair, the points in both pairs are equally distant

Ratio – an interval scale on which an absolute zero is specified. The absolute zero represents the point at which the characteristic being measured is absent.

median The middle point of ordered data. If there are n observations sorted in ascending order, the median refers to the $((n+1)/2)^{th}$ data point.

meta-analysis A statistical synthesis of results from different yet suitably similar studies to produce an overall measurement of effect.

mode The most commonly observed value.

model A simplified description of a system intended to capture the essential features of that system.

modelling The use of mathematical models to elicit relationships between explanatory (independent) and outcome (dependent) variables.

multiple testing When two or more comparisons are made. The problem with multiple testing is that as the number of tests increases, so does the probability of getting a significant result by chance.

negative predictive value The propoportion of negative tests that are truly negative.

normal distribution Also known as the Gaussian distribution. This is the probability distribution of a continuous variable. 'Normal' refers to the fact that it conforms to a rule or norm. The parameters of a normal distribution are the mean and standard deviation; when the mean is 0 and standard deviation is 1, the distribution is called a standardised normal distribution.

null hypothesis The hypothesis that the treatment under investigation is ineffective or shows no difference between groups.

number-needed-to-benefit See number-needed-to-treat.

number-needed-to-harm The number of patients who need to be treated in order to produce one adverse outcome.

number-needed-to-treat The number of patients who need to be treated in order to prevent one adverse outcome.

odds The ratio of the probability of an event occurring to the probability of its not occurring.

odds ratio The ratio of odds in one category of an independent variable to another category that is designated as the reference.

outcome Refers to the result of interest in a study or experiment. There is some degree of uncertainty attached to it.

parameter The value of a characteristic in the population.

population A collection of all the objects or people we are interested in knowing about.

positive predictive value The proportion of positive results that are truly positive.

power The ability of a test to reject the null hypothesis when it is false. Power equals 1 minus type II error.

prevalence The prevalence of a disease is the proportion of a population who are cases at a particular point in time.

probability The frequency of an outcome in the whole population. This is only one of the many ways in which probability can be defined.

probability distribution This refers to the series of probabilities associated with each of the outcomes.

P value The probability of rejecting the null hypothesis when it is in fact true.

quantile A fraction of the distribution if q represents the quantile, the ith value corresponding to q is given by $q \times (n+1)$. If i is not an integer, the value required lies proportionately between the (integer part of i)th value and the next.

random Having no observable pattern.

random effects model meta-analysis A statistical approach to pooling data that assumes random differences between studies and that each study is actually a member of a normally distributed population of studies.

randomisation A method of allocating participants to treatment and control groups so that the characteristics of the participants do not influence the groups to which they are assigned.

randomised-controlled trial Experimental design in which an intervention is compared with another intervention and/or to placebo. Crucially, the allocation of participants to trial groups is randomised.

range The difference between the maximum and the minimum values in the data reference range. See confidence interval.

rank The index of an item in an ordered list.

regression A numerical method to describe the relationship between the outcome variable and one or more predictor variables.

relative frequency The proportion of observations in a sample.

relative risk The ratio of risks in one category of an independent variable to those in another category that is designated as the reference.

risk The probability of an event occurring.

sample The smaller part of the population that we select in order to study and learn more about the population.

sample size calculations A statistical determination of the number of participants who need to complete a study in order reliably to test the hypothesis under investigation. The level of significance, power of the study and minimum acceptable effect size will usually be clearly specified as these are the main factors influencing sample size.

sensitivity A measure of the extent to which a diagnostic test is able to identify true cases.

sensitivity analysis An analysis undertaken to test the influence of a variable or subject on the results. This typically involves analysis with and without the variable or subject in question, with a comparison of the results.

significance level The probability of rejecting a null hypothesis when it is in fact true. The probability is fixed beforehand.

simple random sampling Every member of the population has a known and usually equal probability of being included in the sample.

skewness A measure of symmetry of distribution around the mean. In a symmetrical distribution, skewness is 0.

slope A change in the dependent variable that accompanies a unit change in the independent variable.

specificity The ability of a test to prevent false-positive results.

standard deviation The square root of the variance.

standard error The standard deviation of the distribution of the mean of a sample.

statistic The measurement of an attribute in a sample.

statistics The science of assembling and interpreting numerical data.

statistical inference The process of drawing conclusions from a sample to a wider population.

type I error An error of the first kind whereby the null hypothesis is rejected when it is in fact true. This is usually represented by α.

type II error An error of the second kind whereby the null hypothesis is accepted when it is in fact false. This is usually represented by β.

unbiased estimator An estimator is unbiased if the difference between the true value and the estimated value is zero.

variable A symbolic representation of data. The term implies that its value can vary from observation to observation.

variance The spread of a variable around its mean.

References
and further reading

Main references used

The following books have served as our main references; those wishing to develop a more in-depth appreciation of statistics are advised to consult these core texts. Of the three texts cited, Altman's is perhaps the easiest to engage with, that of Bland also serving as a useful and readable primer. Armitage et al is more complex but is nonetheless a very useful reference text.

Altman DG *Practical Statistics for Medical Research*. London: Chapman & Hall, 1991.

Armitage P Matthews JNS, Berry G *Statistical Methods in Medical Research*. London: Blackwell, 2001.

Bland M *An Introduction to Medical Statistics* (2nd edn). Oxford: Oxford University Press, 1995.

Further reading

Below are listed a number of additional references that we feel are particularly useful to practitioners and researchers wishing to develop further their interests in selected topics covered in this book. To facilitate the most productive use of these texts, we have indicated in square brackets the topics we feel each reference covers best.

Altman DG, Machin D, Bryant TN, Gardner MJ *Statistics with Confidence* (2nd edn). London: BMJ Books, 2000. [Confidence intervals, sample size calculations and the interpretation of diagnostic tests]

Bowers D *Statistics from Scratch. An Introduction for Healthcare Professionals.* Chichester: Wiley, 1996. [Use of the SPSS and EPI-INFO statistical packages]

Brown RA, Swanson Beck J *Medical Statistics on Microcomputers: A Guide to Appropriate Use of Statistical Packages* (2nd edn). London: BMJ Books, 1994. [Use of statistical packages]

Campbell MJ *Statistics at Square Two.* London: BMJ Books, 2001. [Meta-analysis and random effects models]

Campbell MJ, Machin D *Medical Statistics: A Commonsense Approach.* Chichester: Wiley, 1999. [Understanding issues in study design and the use of diagnostic tests]

Chalmers I, Altman DG *Systematic Reviews.* London: BMJ Publishing Group, 1995. [Systematic reviews]

Clayton D, Hills M *Statistical Models in Epidemiology.* Oxford: Oxford University Press, 1993. [Modelling techniques]

Coggon D *Statistics in Clinical Practice.* London: BMJ Books, 1995. [Summarising data]

Colton T *Statistics in Medicine.* Boston: Little, Brown, 1974. [Probability, statistical inference, correlation and regression, and fallacies in numerical reasoning]

Egger M, Davey Smith G, Altman DG *Systematic Reviews in Healthcare: Meta-analysis in Context.* London: BMJ Books, 2001. [Systematic reviews and meta-analysis]

Hill A Bradford *A Short Textbook of Medical Statistics* (11th edn). London: Hodder & Stoughton, 1984. [Statistical evidence and inference]

Last JM *A Dictionary of Epidemiology* (4th edn). Oxford: Oxford University Press, 2001. [Definitions of statistical and epidemiological terms]

Kirkwood BR, Sterne J *Essentials of Medical Statistics.* London: Blackwell, 2003. [Sample size calculations, and discussions on bias and sources of error]

Petrie A, Sabin C *Medical Statistics at a Glance*. Oxford: Blackwell, 2000. [Data entry and the presentation of results]

Pocock SJ *Clinical Trials: A Practical Approach*. Chichester: Wiley, 1983. [Theory and analysis of data from randomised-controlled studies]

Swinscow TDV (revised by Campbell MJ). *Statistics at Square One* (9th edn). London: BMJ Books, 1996. Available online at: http://bmj.com/collections/statsbk/index.shtml [Types of error, and the use of Chi-squared and *t* tests]

Index

Have you found **Basic Skills in Statistics** useful and practical? If so, you may be interested in other books from Class Publishing.

Vital Diabetes
THIRD EDITION £14.99
Dr Charles Fox and Mary MacKinnon

This handy reference guide gives you all the backup you need for best practice in diabetes care, and includes all the vital facts and figures about diabetes for your information and regular use, as well as providing patient and carer information sheets that you can photocopy for patients to take away with them.

'Full of the kind of essential and up-to-date information you need to deliver the best practice in diabetes care.'
M. Carpenter, Diabetes Grapevine

Providing Diabetes Care in General Practice
FOURTH EDITION £24.99
Mary MacKinnon

This practical handbook gives you all the essential information you need to set up and organise health care for people with diabetes in the primary care setting, by allocating tasks to each member of the team. This book also contains clear guidelines for integrating care with the hospital-based services.

'The complete guide for the primary health care team.'
Dr Michael Hall, Chairman of Diabetes UK

Kidney Failure Explained
NEW SECOND EDITION £14.99
Dr Andy Stein and Janet Wild

This fully updated edition of this complete reference manual gives your patients and their families all the information that they could want about managing kidney conditions, and covers every aspect of living with kidney disease – from diagnosis, drugs and treatment, to diet, relationships and sexual relationships.

'This book is, without doubt, the best resource currently available for kidney patients and those who care for them.'
Val Said, kidney transplant patient

Chronic Obstructive Pulmonary Disease in Primary Care
NEW SECOND EDITION £24.99
Dr David Bellamy and Rachel Bellamy

This clear and helpful resource manual addresses the management requirements of GP's and practice nurses. In this book, you will find guidance, protocols, plans and tests – all appropriate to the primary care situation – that will streamline your diagnosis and management of COPD.

'I am sure it will become a classic in the history of COPD Care.'
Duncan Geddes, Professor of Respiratory Medicine and Consultant Physician, Royal Brompton Hospital

PRIORITY ORDER FORM

Cut out or photocopy this form and send it (post free in the UK) to:

Class Publishing Priority Service   **Tel: 01752 202 301**
FREEPOST (PAM 6219)
Plymouth PL6 7ZZ   **Fax: 01752 202 333**

Please send me urgently   *Post included*
(tick boxes below)   *price per copy (UK only)*

☐ **Basic Skills in Statistics**   £17.99
  (ISBN 1 85959 101 9)

☐ **Vital Diabetes**   £17.99
  (ISBN 1 872362 93 1)

☐ **Providing Diabetes Care in General Practice**   £27.99
  (ISBN 1 85959 048 9)

☐ **Kidney Failure Explained**   £17.99
  (ISBN 1 85959 070 5)

☐ **Chronic Obstructive Pulmonary Disease in Primary Care**   £27.99
  (ISBN 1 85959 081 0)

                                          TOTAL _____

Easy ways to pay

Cheque: I enclose a cheque payable to Class Publishing for £ _____
Credit card: Please debit my   ☐ Mastercard   ☐ Visa   ☐ Amex   ☐ Switch

Number _____ Expiry date _____

Name _____

My address for delivery is _____

_____

Town _____ County _____ Postcode _____

Telephone number (in case of query) _____

Credit card billing address if different from above _____

_____

Town _____ County _____ Postcode _____

Class Publishing's guarantee: remember that if, for any reason, you are not satisfied with these books, we will refund all your money, without any questions asked. Prices and VAT rates may be altered for reasons beyond our control.